SINGLE BEST ANSWERS
FOR THE MRCOG PART 2

SINGLE BEST ANSWERS FOR THE MRCOG PART 2

Brian A Magowan FRCOG, DipFetMed
Consultant Obstetrician and Gynaecologist, NHS Borders, Melrose, UK

Mohamed A Otify MSc, MRCOG, DipGynUSS
Specialty Registrar Obstetrics and Gynaecology, South East Scotland, UK

Tarek T El Shamy MBBCH, MSc, MRCOG
Clinical Teaching Fellow, Derby Teaching Hospitals NHS Foundation Trust, Derby, UK

Andrew C Pearson BSc (MedSci)(Hons), DTM&H, MRCOG
Specialty Registrar Obstetrics and Gynaecology, South East Scotland, UK

ELSEVIER

Edinburgh   London   New York   Oxford   Philadelphia   St Louis   Sydney   Toronto 2017

ELSEVIER

ISBN   9780702068812

Notices

Knowledge and best practice in this field are constantly changing. As new research and experience broaden our understanding, changes in research methods, professional practices, or medical treatment may become necessary.

Practitioners and researchers must always rely on their own experience and knowledge in evaluating and using any information, methods, compounds, or experiments described herein. In using such information or methods they should be mindful of their own safety and the safety of others, including parties for whom they have a professional responsibility.

With respect to any drug or pharmaceutical products identified, readers are advised to check the most current information provided (i) on procedures featured or (ii) by the manufacturer of each product to be administered, to verify the recommended dose or formula, the method and duration of administration, and contraindications. It is the responsibility of practitioners, relying on their own experience and knowledge of their patients, to make diagnoses, to determine dosages and the best treatment for each individual patient, and to take all appropriate safety precautions.

To the fullest extent of the law, neither the publisher nor the authors, contributors, or editors, assume any liability for any injury and/or damage to persons or property as a matter of products liability, negligence or otherwise, or from any use or operation of any methods, products, instructions, or ideas contained in the material herein.

Content Strategist: Pauline Graham
Content Development Specialist: Helen Leng
Project Manager: Louisa Talbott
Designer: Christian Bilbow
Illustration: Graphic World, Inc. and Matrix Art Services

Printed in China

Last digit is the print number: 9   8   7   6   5   4   3   2   1

Contents

Modules

The RCOG core speciality training curriculum is divided into 19 modules and the questions are arranged to match these subject areas. All of these, with the exception of Module 4 (Ethics and Legal Issues) and Module 19 (Developing Professionalism), are examinable in the MRCOG Part 2.

Preface

The MRCOG Part 2 is one of the toughest postgraduate membership exams and, even with the best preparation, failure is common. This is especially true for those practising outside the UK and Ireland for whom certain practices or procedures, or even simply abbreviations, may be unfamiliar.

This book aims to help in two ways. The first, of course, is to practise answering single-best-answer (SBA) questions. The second is to provide a break in the endless reading and memorising required. As each answer is accompanied by a concise explanation and reference, learning points can be quickly absorbed; this is not the time for 'self-directed learning' – your time is precious and we aim to give you as much learning as possible on a big silver spoon!

Many of these questions are at the more difficult end of the SBA spectrum. This is intentional, as the exam is intended to explore some of the more complex issues in our speciality. It is also, therefore, likely that you will disagree with some of our answers. This could be because we have made an error, and for this we apologize, although errors occasionally appear in the actual exam as well. It might also be because some new research or guidelines have been published but, as the answers are clearly referenced, you can identify this quickly and move on. Most commonly, however, it will be because clinical practice at this level is full of uncertainties, and balancing these carefully has some element of individuality. We hope, however, that our justifications will add to your learning and preparation, and will help to continue preparing you for excellence in clinical practice.

You will not have reached this stage in your career without some knowledge of passing exams. This exam, however, is a big one and we would be delighted if this book is able to provide a useful springboard to clearing a very worthwhile hurdle in this challenging, but hugely rewarding, speciality.

AP, MO, TES, BM

Abbreviations

A&E: Accident and Emergency
ACE: angiotensin-converting enzyme
AFP: alpha-fetoprotein
AKI: acute kidney injury
BMI: body mass index
BP: blood pressure
bpm: beats per minute
BSO: bilateral salpingo-oophorectomy
CBT: cognitive behavioural therapy
CI: chief investigator
CIN: cervical intraepithelial neoplasia
COCP: combined oral contraceptive pill
CRL: crown rump length
CRP: C-reactive protein
CSF: cerebrospinal fluid
CTG: cardiotocography
CTPA: computed tomographic pulmonary angiography
CXR: chest x-ray
DES: diethylstilboestrol
DMPA: depot medroxyprogesterone acetate
DV: ductus venosus
DVP: deepest vertical pool
ECG: electrocardiogram
ECV: external cephalic version
FBC: full blood count
FDA: Food and Drug Administration
FIGO: International Federation of Gynaecology and Obstetrics
FRAX: fracture risk assessment
FSH: follicle-stimulating hormone
GCT: germ cell tumour
GnRH: gonadotropin-releasing hormone
GP: general practitioner

HIV: human immunodeficiency virus
hMG: human menopausal gonadotropins
HPV: human papillomavirus
HRT: hormone replacement therapy
HSG: hysterosalpingogram
HyCoSy: hysterosalpingo-contrast sonography
ICSI: intracytoplasmic sperm injection
Ig: immunoglobulin
IOTA: International Ovarian Tumour Analysis Group
IUCD: intrauterine contraceptive device
IUD: intrauterine device
IUFD: intrauterine fetal demise
IUI: intrauterine insemination
IUS: intrauterine system
IV: intravenous
IVF: in vitro fertilization
LCI: local chief investigator
LDH: lactate dehydrogenase
LFT: liver function tests
LH: luteinizing hormone
LIF: left iliac fossa
LMWH: low molecular weight heparin
LNG-IUS: levonorgestrel intrauterine system
MCA: middle cerebral artery
NICE: National Institute for Health and Care Excellence
OA: occiput anterior
OHSS: ovarian hyperstimulation syndrome
OP: occiput posterior
PCOS: polycystic ovary syndrome
PCR: protein/creatinine ratio
PDS: polydioxanone suture
PE: pulmonary embolism

PI: principal investigator

PID: pelvic inflammatory disease

PPH: postpartum haemorrhage

PV: per vaginam

RAADP: routine antenatal anti-D immunoglobulin prophylaxis

RCOG: Royal College of Obstetricians and Gynaecologists

RCT: randomized controlled trial

Rh: Rhesus

RMI: risk of malignancy index

RRBSO: risk-reducing bilateral salpingo-oophorectomy

SFH: symphysis fundal height

SGA: small-for-gestational-age

SHBG: sex hormone-binding hormone

SIRS: systemic inflammatory response syndrome

SSRI: selective serotonin reuptake inhibitor

STAN: ST analysis

STI: sexually transmitted infection

SVD: spontaneous vaginal delivery

TAH: total abdominal hysterectomy

TRAP: twin reversed arterial perfusion

TSH: thyroid-stimulating hormone

TTTS: twin-to-twin transfusion syndrome

TVT: tension-free vaginal tape

U&E: urea and electrolytes

UA: umbilical artery

UAE: uterine artery embolization

UFH: unfractionated heparin

UKMEC: UK Medical Eligibility Criteria

VTE: venous thromboembolism

WBC: white blood cell count

QUESTIONS

1. You see a 24-year-old woman in your antenatal clinic. She is at 11 weeks' gestation in her first pregnancy and is known to have epilepsy controlled with lamotrigine. On the Internet she has noticed that it is a FDA Category C drug.

What does this mean?

Options

A. Animal reproduction studies have shown an adverse effect on the fetus, and there are no adequate and well-controlled studies in humans, but potential benefits may warrant the use of the drug in pregnant women despite potential risks.

B. Adequate and well-controlled studies have failed to demonstrate a risk to the fetus in the first trimester of pregnancy (and there is no evidence of risk in later trimesters).

C. Animal reproduction studies have failed to demonstrate a risk to the fetus, and there are no adequate and well-controlled studies in pregnant women.

D. There is positive evidence of human fetal risk based on adverse reaction data from investigational or marketing experience or studies in humans, but potential benefits may warrant use of the drug in pregnant women despite potential risks.

E. Studies in animals or humans have demonstrated fetal abnormalities and/or there is positive evidence of human fetal risk based on adverse reaction data from investigational or marketing experience, and the risks involved in the use of the drug in pregnant women clearly outweigh potential benefits.

2. Lord Fraser, in his ruling of the Gillick case in the House of Lords, produced guidelines regarding contraceptive advice given by doctors. Doctors can proceed to advise and give contraception provided they are satisfied with four of the following five criteria.

Which one does not apply?

Options

    A. The girl (although under 16 years of age) will understand advice.

    B. The doctor cannot persuade her to inform her parents or to allow the parents to be informed that she is seeking contraceptive advice.

    C. She is very likely to continue having sexual intercourse with or without contraceptive treatment.

    D. Unless she receives contraceptive advice or treatment her physical or mental health or both are likely to suffer.

    E. Her best interests require the doctor to give her contraceptive advice, treatment or both, but only with the parental consent.

3. A 25-year-old para 2 at 30 weeks' gestation presents to your day assessment unit with right-sided loin pain and feeling generally unwell. On examination her temperature is 38°C, pulse rate 90 bpm, respiratory rate 20 per minute and BP 110/70 mm Hg. There is right-sided renal angle tenderness. Urinalysis shows 2+ blood, 3+ leucocytes, 2+ protein and 1+ nitrite. The ST1 doctor, who is about to go home, prescribes cefuroxime and metronidazole without checking if she is allergic to any antibiotics. The pharmacist is too busy to check the drug chart. The bank midwife is busy as well and gives the antibiotics without having them checked with another midwife. The patient is given the antibiotics and develops an allergic reaction.

Which of the following is the correct combination of causal factors for this error?

Options

    A. Poor leadership and poor teamwork.

    B. Poor teamwork and circumventing safe systems.

    C. Poor teamwork and correct equipment not available.

    D. Poor leadership and not following emergency procedures.

    E. Circumventing safe systems and not following safe procedures.

4. You see a 22-year-old woman in your gynaecology clinic who presents with pelvic pain and dyspareunia for 7 months. She is worried that she may have an ovarian cyst. Her mother was diagnosed recently with ovarian cancer. You offer to perform a bimanual examination to rule out adnexal pathology.

What is the accuracy rate of pelvic examination performed by an experienced gynaecologist in detecting adnexal masses?

Options

   A. Around 10%.
   B. Around 30%.
   C. Around 50%.
   D. Around 70%.
   E. Around 90%.

5. You are the on-call registrar when the gynaecology ward sister asks you to see a 55-year-old patient and her husband. She had undergone a laparotomy earlier in the day and had unexpectedly been found to have 'inoperable advanced ovarian cancer'. The couple asks you about the operative findings and you decide to break the bad news.

What is the next most important step before breaking the bad news?

Options

   A. Give a warning shot.
   B. Identify the couple's main concern.
   C. Hand your bleep to the nurse and make sure you are not interrupted.
   D. Maintain eye contact.
   E. Prepare yourself.

ANSWERS

1. Answer: A.

Explanation: U.S. FDA classification system for drugs used in pregnancy. Answer A is Category C, B is Category A, C is Category B and answers D and E are Category D and E, respectively.

Reference: Chan M, Wong ICK, Sutcliffe AG (2012). Prescription drug use in pregnancy: more evidence of safety is needed. *The Obstetrician & Gynaecologist* 14, 87–92.

2. Answer: E.

Explanation: The judgment states that 'Her best interests require the doctor to give her contraceptive advice, treatment or both without the parental consent'.

Reference: Jha S, Rowland S (2014). Litigation in gynaecology. *The Obstetrician & Gynaecologist* 16, 51–57.

3. Answer: B.

Explanation: In this scenario there are two causal factors: (1) poor teamwork and (2) circumventing safe systems. If an organization has a weak safety culture, there are many opportunities for errors to occur. In this case both the midwife and the pharmacist circumvented safe systems, which may become a common practice when established guidelines are not followed.

Reference: Industrial Psychology Research Centre (2012). ANTS: a behavioural marker system for rating anaesthetists' nontechnical skills. Available at: http://www.abdn.ac.uk/iprc/ants.

4. Answer: D.

Explanation: In a prospective cohort study, the overall pelvic examination was accurate 70.2% of the time for attending physicians, 64.0% for residents and 57.3% for medical students. Postgraduate years of experience seemed to improve the likelihood of identifying adnexal masses. When attending physicians described an adnexal mass by examination, the chances of finding one at surgery were five times greater than not finding one.

Reference: Padilla LA, Radosevich DM, Milad MP (2005). Limitations of the pelvic examination for evaluation of the female pelvic organs. *International Journal of Gynecology & Obstetrics* 88 (1), 84–88.

5. Answer: E.

Explanation: Before seeing the patient, it is essential to be familiar with the case record and all relevant information to be discussed, especially if you have not always been the doctor caring for the woman.

Reference: Kaye P (1996). *Breaking Bad News: A 10-Step Approach*. Northampton: EPL Publications.

Module 2 Teaching, appraisal and assessment

QUESTIONS

6. You are asked to teach gynaecologic emergencies at the emergency department monthly teaching. Unfortunately you have not been able to ascertain the grade or level of previous gynaecology experience of those who are attending. You start by getting the casualty doctors to discuss basic pelvic anatomy and then the basics of early pregnancy. Next you base the level of your further teaching on the level of knowledge they displayed in these initial basic subjects.

What would best describe this teaching method?

Options

    A. Brainstorming.
    B. Delphi technique.
    C. Fish bowl.
    D. Problem-based learning.
    E. Snowballing.

7. A ST1 colleague is confused at the array of assessments available in the electronic training portfolio and asks you which are formative and which are summative.

Which of the following is an example of a formative assessment?

Options

    A. ARCP.
    B. MRCOG Part 1.
    C. MRCOG Part 2.
    D. MRCOG Part 3.
    E. TO1.

8. A consultant is finding it cumbersome preparing for an appraisal.

How frequently should the appraisal normally take place?

Options

    A. Annually.
    B. Biannually.
    C. Every 3 years.
    D. Every 5 years.
    E. Every 10 years.

Module 2 Teaching, appraisal and assessment

ANSWERS

6. Answer: E.

Explanation: Formal names have been developed for many commonly used teaching methods. Brainstorming is spontaneous group discussion to produce ideas and ways of solving a problem. In the Delphi technique each person provides anonymous answers and a facilitator amalgamates the results for feedback. The fish bowl method is a small group-teaching technique in which a number of students engage in a discussion while observers form a circle around them. In problem-based learning, learners are given a problem or case to discuss; using self-directed learning they are encouraged to identify and research their own learning objectives.

Reference: Duthie SJ, Garden AS (2010). The teacher, the learner and the method. *The Obstetrician & Gynaecologist* 12, 273–280.

7. Answer E.

Explanation: TO1 is a feedback form sent to a colleague as a part of multisource feedback. The specialist trainee's supervisor will then compile these together to make a TO2 which will provide feedback to the trainee. The others are all summative (i.e., they have a pass/fail or grade). In the ARCP (annual review of competency progression) the specialty trainee is assessed against the matrix of educational progression to assess whether or not they can progress to the next year of training. The MRCOG exams are pass/fail exams (as you will be well aware!) UK training now has large amounts of administrative requirements and tasks to perform, and this is accompanied by a large bulk of technical jargon and acronyms. Overseas candidates would be well advised to spend some time familiarizing themselves with these.

Reference: Royal College of Obstetricians and Gynaecologists. StratOG, eLearning, core training.

8. Answer: A.

Explanation: Appraisal should take place annually as part of a five-year revalidation cycle.

Reference: Royal College of Obstetricians and Gynaecologists. StratOG, core training, The General Medical Council, good medical practice.

Module 3 Information technology, clinical governance and research

QUESTIONS

9. Your hospital is taking part in a large multicentre clinical trial into the management of reduced fetal movements. One of your consultants is the nominated lead for the conduct of the trial in your hospital.

What is the name of the consultant's role?

Options

    A. Chief investigator.
    B. Local chief investigator.
    C. Principal investigator.
    D. Sponsor.
    E. Supervising investigator.

10. A RCOG Green-top Guideline makes a recommendation based on a well-conducted systematic review of RCTs. The evidence is directly applicable to the target population of the recommendation.

What is the classification of this level of evidence?

Options

    A. 1++.
    B. 1+.
    C. 1−.
    D. A.
    E. B.

11. A new serum marker, XZT, is being assessed to see if it is helpful in PE to a safe level in pregnant women. In nonpregnant women a negative XZT has been shown to have a high negative predictive value for PE. CTPA is used as the gold standard. The 998 pregnant women having a CTPA performed to assess for PE have their XZT checked. Forty-eight of the women are diagnosed with PE based on CTPA; of these, 47 have a positive XZT and one has a negative XZT. Over 950 women have no PE diagnosed on CTPA; of these, 100 have a positive XZT and 850 have a negative XZT.

What is the negative predictive value of XZT for PE in this population of pregnant women?

Options

  A. 89.9%.
  B. 93.9%.
  C. 95%.
  D. 97.9%.
  E. 99.9%.

12. A study looks to compare the birth weight of the 140 babies delivered by forceps with the 1724 delivered by SVD in a year on a labour ward.

What would be the most suitable statistical test to use in this comparison?

Options

  A. Analysis of variance.
  B. Friedman test.
  C. Paired t-test.
  D. Pearson correlation coefficient.
  E. Unpaired t-test.

13. The operating department of your hospital runs a teaching day on human factors.

Which is a Department of Health 'Never Event'?

Options

  A. A healthy 25 year old is diagnosed with breech presentation at 37 weeks' gestation. She declines ECV and agrees to elective caesarean section, which is booked for 39^{+2} weeks. She spontaneously labours in the night at 38^{+6} weeks' gestation, and on arrival is found to be 3 cm dilated with regular contractions. A caesarean section is performed. There is extension into the right uterine angle and unexpected hypotonicity. The ST1 performing the caesarean section desperately, but unfruitfully, attempts to get haemostasis. She appears to lose her situational awareness and refuses to seek assistance. The theatre sister and anaesthetist agree to summon help, but unfortunately the ST5 is dealing with a major PPH in the labour ward. The consultant is summoned from home but his car breaks down, delaying his arrival. Extensive blood products are used, but the resuscitation efforts cannot keep up with the haemorrhage. The surgical ST5 comes to help, but the patient has a cardiac arrest on the operating table while he is scrubbing. After 60 minutes of cardiopulmonary resuscitation (CPR) a decision is made to stop.

B. A laparoscopic BSO is performed for ovarian torsion in a 57-year-old woman. After removing the second affected ovary from the abdomen, the operator goes to remove the healthy ovary which he has left in the pelvis after earlier removal for later retrieval. The ovary cannot be found and, after 30 minutes of searching laparoscopically, it is decided that laparotomy would be of greater harm than benefit.

C. A patient is diagnosed with a left-sided ectopic pregnancy and is consented for a left salpingectomy. At laparoscopy, the ectopic is on the right side and the right tube is removed.

D. A 33-year-old para 4 (four previous caesarean sections) undergoes elective caesarean section. A placenta accreta is found; the surgeon tries to remove the placenta firmly and tears it. Bleeding is catastrophic and, despite excellent resuscitation efforts and a caesarean hysterectomy, the woman dies. Later the antenatal care is criticized for not looking more closely at the placenta on the 20-week scan.

E. A 37-year-old morbidly obese para (previous spontaneous vaginal deliveries) undergoes elective caesarean section for breech presentation. The uterine incision extends into the angle and there is severe hypotonicity. Despite surgical salvage and anaesthetic resuscitation she bleeds catastrophically, quicker than blood can be replaced. She has an asystolic cardiac arrest on the operating table, and resuscitation attempts fail.

ANSWERS

9. Answer: C.

Explanation: The PI is the authorized healthcare professional responsible for the conduct of the trial in a particular site. The CI has the overall responsibility for the trial. The sponsor takes responsibility for the initiation, conduct and financial arrangements of the clinical study (this can be an institution, company or person).

Reference: Thangaratinam S, Khan K (2015). Participation in research as a means of improving quality of care: the role of a principal investigator in multicentre clinical trials. *The Obstetrician & Gynaecologist* 17 (1), 55–61.

10. Answer: B.

Explanation: This well-conducted systematic review of RCTs is level 1+ evidence. The recommendation would be grade A.

Reference: Royal College of Obstetricians and Gynaecologists (2006). *Development of RCOG Green-top Guidelines: policies and processes.* Clinical Governance Advice No. 1a, 2nd ed. London: RCOG.

11. Answer: E.

Explanation: The 850 women that have a negative XZT do not have a PE (presuming CTPA is the gold standard), and one of those with a negative XZT will have a PE. Negative predictive value is the probability that subjects with a negative test truly do not have the disease: 850/851 = 0.998 = approximately 99.9%. You will not have a calculator in the examination but will be expected to perform basic mathematical functions. It may be helpful to round the numbers to perform an approximate calculation to use to pick the best answer.

Reference: Royal College of Obstetricians and Gynaecologists. StratOG, core training, the obstetrician and gynaecologist as a teacher and researcher.

12. Answer: E.

Explanation: This is a comparison of biological variables within large samples, so the population can be assumed to be parametric. There are two separate groups, so it is an unpaired *t*-test. If there was one group (e.g. the weight of the babies on days 1 and 5) it would be a paired *t*-test. Because performing multiple unpaired *t*-tests would result in an increased chance of committing a statistical type I error, analysis of variance tests (ANOVAs) are useful in comparing (testing) three or more means (groups or variables) for statistical significance (the Friedman test can be used for this with nonparametric data). The Pearson correlation coefficient is a measure of the strength of the linear relationship between two variables (the nonparametric equivalent is the Spearman Rank correlation coefficient).

References: Royal College of Obstetricians and Gynaecologists. StratOG, core training, the obstetrician and gynaecologist as a teacher and researcher.
Scally AJ (2014). A practical introduction to medical statistics. *The Obstetrician & Gynaecologist* 16(2), 121–128.

13. Answer: E.

Explanation: A maternal death from PPH at scheduled caesarean section is a Department of Health 'Never Event'. Exclusions are placenta accreta, maternal preexisting bleeding disorder or maternal refusal of blood. In the case in A it is not a scheduled caesarean section. Never Events are serious and largely preventable patient safety incidents that should not occur if the available preventative measures have been implemented by healthcare providers. Just because a case is not classified as a Never Event does not mean that preventable errors have not occurred.

The ectopic case is not an example of wrong-site surgery, although certainly it would have been sensible for the consent form not to specify the side (contrast from, for example, a limb amputation, so this rationale for not specifying the side will often need to be explained to theatre staff who are unfamiliar with gynaecologic procedures). The ovary is not a foreign object, so this is no foreign object retention.

References: Macdonald M, Gosakan R, Cooper A, Fothergill D (2014). *The Obstetrician & Gynaecologist* 16 (2), 109–114.

NHS England, Patient safety, Never Events. https://www.england.nhs.uk/patientsafety/never-events.

Modules 5 and 6
Core surgical skills and postoperative care

QUESTIONS

14. A 31-year-old para 1 undergoes radical vaginal trachelectomy and laparoscopic bilateral lymph node dissection for early cervical cancer. She presents with paraesthesia over the mons pubis, labia majora and the femoral triangle.

Her symptoms are most likely caused by injury to which of the following?

Options

    A. Lateral cutaneous nerve.
    B. Genitofemoral nerve.
    C. Ilioinguinal nerve.
    D. Femoral nerve.
    E. Pudendal nerve.

15. A 57-year-old para 4 undergoes vaginal hysterectomy and sacrospinous ligament fixation. She complains of postoperative gluteal pain that worsens in the seated position.

Her symptoms are most likely caused by injury to which of the following?

Options

    A. Lateral cutaneous nerve.
    B. Genitofemoral nerve.
    C. Ilioinguinal nerve.
    D. Pudendal nerve.
    E. Femoral nerve.

16. The enhanced recovery approach to preoperative, perioperative and postoperative care has major benefits for many patients in relation to quicker recovery following major surgery. It facilitates shorter hospital stay with no increase in readmission rates. This has clear benefits for patients and their families and for healthcare services.

Which of the following is not a component of the enhanced recovery pathways?

Options

A. Optimized preoperative haemoglobin level.
B. Avoidance of carbohydrate loading.
C. Use of regional blocks.
D. Minimal-access surgery.
E. Avoidance of systemic opiates.

17. A 65-year-old diabetic patient with a BMI of 35 kg/m^2 had a TAH+BSO for complex endometrial hyperplasia with atypia.

What is the best pharmacologic thromboprophylaxis regimen for this patient?

Options

A. LMWH for 7 days.
B. LMWH for 28 days.
C. LMWH while an inpatient.
D. UFH while an inpatient.
E. Pharmacologic thromboprophylaxis only if additional risk for VTE.

18. Myomectomy for large uterine fibroids can be associated with massive blood loss, blood transfusion and conversion from myomectomy to hysterectomy.

Which of the following is not a recognized intervention to reduce blood loss at the time of open myomectomy?

Options

A. Preoperative GnRH analogues.
B. Uterine artery tourniquet.
C. Intramyometrial vasopressin.
D. Tranexamic acid.
E. Oxytocin.

19. You are asked to prepare a talk for your colleagues on laparoscopic electrosurgical complications.

Which of the following is not one of the safety measures to prevent such laparoscopic complications?

Options

    A. Inspect insulation carefully before use.
    B. Use the lowest possible effective power setting.
    C. Do not activate in close proximity to another instrument.
    D. Use a high-voltage waveform for monopolar diathermy (cut).
    E. Use brief intermittent activation.

20. The Smead–Jones closure is a mass closure technique of the anterior abdominal wall using a far–far, near–near approach. The closure is performed using a delayed absorbable suture to include all the abdominal wall structures on the far–far portion and only the anterior fascia on the near–near portion. This allows good healing without intervening fat or muscle.

Which of the following best describes the rate of fascial dehiscence with running mass closure of the abdomen?

Options

    A. 0.04%.
    B. 0.4%.
    C. 4%.
    D. 14%.
    E. 24%.

21. You are assisting your consultant in a Burch colposuspension procedure for urodynamic stress incontinence after an unsuccessful TVT procedure.

Which of the following transverse skin incisions allows the easiest access to the space of Retzius?

Options

    A. Pfannenstiel incision.
    B. Kustner incision.

    C. Cherney incision.
    D. Maylard incision.
    E. Joel–Cohen incision.

22. A 39-year-old para 2 presents with an 8-month history of pelvic pain. She has a previous vertical abdominal incision for a ruptured appendix and undergoes a diagnostic laparoscopy using closed-entry technique at Palmer's point.

Which of the following describes the correct anatomic position of Palmer's point?

Options

    A. 3 cm below the left costal margin in the midclavicular line.
    B. 3 cm below the left costal margin in the midaxillary line.
    C. 3 cm below the right costal margin in the midclavicular line.
    D. 3 cm below the right costal margin in the midaxillary line.
    E. 3 cm above the symphysis pubis in the midline.

23. You are asked to see a 49-year-old patient in the emergency department who is day 9 following a TAH for multiple uterine fibroids. She presents feeling unwell and has lower abdominal pain. Her bowels have been opening regularly and she has had no bloating, nausea or vomiting. On examination her pulse rate is 92 bpm, BP 110/70 mm Hg, temperature 38°C and respiratory rate of 20 per minute. Urinalysis is clear. The wound is erythematous, indurated and tender to touch. Her haemoglobin is 100 g/L, WBC is 15×10^9/L and CRP of 50 mg/L.

What is the most likely diagnosis?

Options

    A. Sepsis.
    B. Septic shock.
    C. SIRS
    D. Bacteraemia.
    E. Toxic shock syndrome.

24. You see a 28-year-old woman in your clinic. She is referred by her GP with a 6-month history of chronic pelvic pain and deep dyspareunia. A pelvic ultrasound scan shows a retroverted uterus, 4 cm endometrioma on the right ovary, normal left ovary and no free fluid in the pelvis. She is using the progesterone-only pill for contraception, and this has helped slightly with the pain. You consent her for laparoscopy and ovarian cystectomy and discuss risks and potential complications associated with these.

Which of the following best describes the risk of bowel injury?

Options

    A. 15% of bowel injuries might not be diagnosed at the time of laparoscopy.

    B. 25% of bowel injuries might not be diagnosed at the time of laparoscopy.

    C. 35% of bowel injuries might not be diagnosed at the time of laparoscopy.

    D. 45% of bowel injuries might not be diagnosed at the time of laparoscopy.

    E. 55% of bowel injuries might not be diagnosed at the time of laparoscopy.

25. You see a 42-year-old woman in your gynaecology clinic. She presents with a history of heavy periods and is up to date with her smears. There is no postcoital bleeding. Pelvic ultrasound on the second day of her menstrual cycle shows a bulky uterus with a small, well-defined hyperechoic mass in the endometrial cavity. A feeding vessel extending to the mass is noted on colour Doppler imaging and both ovaries are unremarkable. The appearances are suggestive of an endometrial polyp. You consent her for diagnostic hysteroscopy, endometrial polypectomy and insertion of LNG-IUS.

What is the risk of damage to the uterus?

Options

    A. Very common (1/1–1/10).

    B. Common (1/10–1/100).

    C. Uncommon (1/100–1/1000).

D. Rare (1/1000–1/10000).
E. Very rare (less than 1/10000).

26. You see a 45-year-old African-Caribbean woman in your clinic who presents with a large, painless abdominal swelling for 12 months and reports urinary frequency but no dysuria. There is no change in her bowel pattern. Her cycle is 5/28 with passage of blood clots and flooding. She has completed her family and is up to date with her smears. On examination, her abdomen is distended and palpates an irregular and firm mobile nontender pelviabdominal mass equivalent to a 28-week-sized pregnancy. On bimanual examination it is not possible to palpate the uterus separate from this mass. Abdominal and pelvic ultrasound scan suggests multiple uterine fibroids, the largest of which is intramural and measures $14 \times 12 \times 10$ cm. Both ovaries are unremarkable. You discuss abdominal hysterectomy with her and she tells you she wants to keep her cervix.

What is the rate for residual stump cancer of the cervix?

Options

A. 0.003%.
B. 0.03%.
C. 0.3%.
D. 3%.
E. 30%.

27. You are asked to see a 21-year-old para 1 in the early pregnancy assessment unit. She is 9 weeks into her second pregnancy and presents with cramping abdominal pain and vaginal bleeding. Pelvic ultrasound scan shows a picture of incomplete miscarriage. She opts for surgical management of the miscarriage, and you consent her for surgical evacuation.

What is the risk of uterine perforation at the time of surgical evacuation?

Options

A. 0.005%.
B. 0.05%.

C. 0.5%.

D. 5%.

E. 50%.

28. You have been asked by your consultant to write a patient information leaflet on caesarean section. You decide to include information on serious and frequently occurring risks.

What is the incidence of ureteric injury at the time of caesarean section?

Options

A. 0.003%.

B. 0.03%.

C. 0.3%.

D. 3%.

E. 30%.

29. You are performing a diagnostic laparoscopy for a 31-year-old para 1 with a 10-month history of pelvic pain. You attempt insertion of the Veress needle twice. The intra-abdominal pressure is 15 mm Hg.

What is your most appropriate next step?

Options

A. Proceed with pneumoperitoneum.

B. Proceed with laparotomy.

C. Proceed with direct trocar insertion.

D. Proceed with third attempt.

E. Proceed with Palmer's point entry.

30. You perform laparoscopy for a 27-year-old para 2 with a 6 × 5 × 7 cm left ovarian dermoid cyst. She has had two previous caesarean sections. You use closed-entry technique and insufflate the abdomen to 25 mm Hg before inserting the primary trocar in the umbilicus. After introducing the laparoscope you suspect that a loop of bowel is adherent to the anterior abdominal wall at the primary port site.

What is your most appropriate next step?

Options

    A. Proceed with laparotomy.
    B. Visualize the primary trocar site from a secondary port.
    C. Continue with planned procedure.
    D. Call the general surgeon.
    E. Reinsert the primary port in Palmer's point.

31. You are assisting in a total laparoscopic hysterectomy and BSO for extensive endometriosis. The left ureter is accidentally transected at the time of coagulation and division of the uterine artery.

What is the most appropriate intervention?

Options

    A. Ureteroureterostomy.
    B. Transureteroureterostomy.
    C. Ureteroneocystostomy.
    D. Percutaneous nephrostomy.
    E. Ureteric stent.

32. You are performing a hysteroscopy and endometrial biopsy on a 65-year-old para 3 who presents with postmenopausal bleeding and a 9-mm-thick endometrium. You manage to dilate the cervix but there is sudden loss of resistance. You suspect uterine perforation, introduce a 5-mm hysteroscope and recognize a hole on the anterior uterine wall.

What is the most appropriate immediate intervention?

Options

    A. Alert team, IV antibiotics and observe.
    B. Call the general surgeon.
    C. Proceed with diagnostic laparoscopy.
    D. Proceed with laparotomy.
    E. Arrange for a CXR looking for air under diaphragm.

33. You see a 75-year-old patient who had an abdominal hysterectomy 2 days previously. She complains of muscle weakness, palpitations and paraesthesia, and she is oliguric. An ECG shows loss of P-waves, wide QRS complexes and peaked T-waves. The K^+ level is 6.3 mmol/L.

What is the most appropriate immediate intervention?

Options

- A. IV 10 ml 10% calcium gluconate over 2 to 5 minutes.
- B. 10 IU fast-acting insulin (Actrapid) added to 50 ml of 50% dextrose infused IV over 20 minutes.
- C. 5 mg salbutamol nebulizer.
- D. Stat 500 ml bolus of Hartmann's solution IVI.
- E. Stop any drugs that contain potassium.

ANSWERS

14. Answer: B.

Explanation: The genitofemoral nerve (L1–L2) transverses the anterior surface of psoas and lies immediately lateral to the external iliac vessels. It divides into a genital branch, which enters the deep inguinal ring, and a femoral branch, which passes deep to the inguinal ligament within the femoral sheath. This nerve is susceptible to injury during pelvic sidewall surgery and during removal of the external iliac nodes. Genitofemoral nerve injury results in paraesthesia over the mons pubis, labia majora and femoral triangle.

Reference: Kuponiyi O, Alleemudder DI, Latunde-Dada A, Eedarapalli P (2014). Nerve injuries associated with gynaecological surgery. *The Obstetrician & Gynaecologist* 16, 29–36.

15. Answer: D.

Explanation: The pudendal nerve (S2–S4) exits the pelvis initially through the greater sciatic foramen below the piriformis. Importantly, it runs behind the lateral third of the sacrospinous ligament and ischial spine alongside the internal pudendal artery and immediately reenters the pelvis through the lesser sciatic foramen to the pudendal canal (Alcock's canal). This nerve is susceptible to entrapment injuries during sacrospinous ligament fixation, because it runs behind the lateral aspect of the sacrospinous ligament.

Reference: Kuponiyi O, Alleemudder DI, Latunde-Dada A, Eedarapalli P (2014). Nerve injuries associated with gynaecological surgery. *The Obstetrician & Gynaecologist* 16, 29–36.

16. Answer: B.

Explanation: The use of complex carbohydrate drinks has been shown to be beneficial in colorectal surgery.

Reference: Torbre E, Crawford R, Nordin A, Acheson N (2013). Enhanced recovery in gynaecology. *The Obstetrician & Gynaecologist* 15, 263–268.

17. Answer: A.

Explanation: If the VTE risk is increased, mechanical VTE prophylaxis should be offered at admission and continued until mobility is no longer significantly reduced. If the risk of major bleeding is low, LMWH (or UFH for patients with severe renal impairment or established renal failure) should be added until mobility is no longer significantly reduced (generally 5–7 days). If major cancer surgery in the abdomen or pelvis is performed, pharmacologic prophylaxis should be continued for 28 days after surgery.

Reference: The National Institute for Health and Care Excellence (2010). Venous thromboembolism–reducing the risk. London.

18. Answer: E.

Explanation: There is no benefit from using oxytocin during myomectomy, because there are few myometrial oxytocin receptors outside pregnancy.

Reference: Shepherd JH, Marcus E (2011). *Shaw's Textbook of Operative Gynaecology*, 7th ed. India: Elsevier.

19. Answer: D.

Explanation: Low-voltage waveform for monopolar diathermy (cut) should be used to avoid complications.

Reference: Minas V, Gul N, Aust T, Doyle M, Rowlands D (2014). Urinary tract injuries in laparoscopic gynaecologic surgery; prevention, recognition and management. *The Obstetrician & Gynaecologist* 16, 19–28.

20. Answer: B.

Explanation: The fascial dehiscence rate with running mass closure of the abdomen is 0.4%.

Reference: Raghavan R, Arya P, Arya P, China S (2014). Abdominal incisions and sutures in obstetrics and gynaecology. *The Obstetrician & Gynaecologist* 16, 13–18.

21. Answer: C.

Explanation: The Cherney incision involves transection of the rectus muscles at their insertion on the pubic symphysis and retraction cephalad to improve exposure. This can be used for urinary incontinence procedures to access the space of Retzius and to gain exposure to the pelvic sidewall for hypogastric artery ligation.

Reference: Raghavan R, Arya P, Arya P, China S (2014). Abdominal incisions and sutures in obstetrics and gynaecology. *The Obstetrician & Gynaecologist* 16, 13–18.

22. Answer: A.

Explanation: Palmer's point is situated in the left midclavicular line 3 cm below the costal margin. The left upper quadrant is the area where adhesions are least likely to be found following previous surgery, except where the surgery was specifically performed in this area as for a splenectomy.

Reference: Frappell J (2012). Laparoscopic entry after previous surgery. *The Obstetrician & Gynaecologist* 14, 207–209.

23. Answer: A.

Explanation: A diagnosis of SIRS is made if any two of the following criteria are met:
- Temperature greater than 38.3°C or less than 36°C.
- Respiratory rate greater than 20 per minute or $PaCO_2$ less than 32 mm Hg (4.3 kPa).
- Heart rate greater than 90 bpm.
- Total white cell count less than $4 \times 10^9/L$ or greater than $12 \times 10^9/L$.

A diagnosis of sepsis is made if there is a diagnosis of SIRS in the presence of an infection. This becomes severe sepsis if there is sepsis together with evidence of organ dysfunction. Septic shock is said to occur when there is sepsis associated with hypotension (systolic BP less than 90 mm Hg or a reduction of greater than 40 mm Hg from baseline) or lactic acidosis (lactate greater than 4 mmol/L) despite adequate fluid resuscitation.

Reference: Soong J, Soni N (2012). Sepsis: Recognition and treatment. *Clinical Medicine* 12, 276–280.

24. Answer: A.

Explanation: Damage to bowel, bladder, uterus or major blood vessels which would require immediate repair by laparoscopy or laparotomy is uncommon. However, around 15% of bowel injuries might not be diagnosed at the time of laparoscopy.

Reference: Royal College of Obstetricians and Gynaecologists (2008). Diagnostic laparoscopy. Consent Advice No. 2. London.

25. Answer: C.

Explanation: Damage to the uterus is uncommon, and this is defined as between 1/100 and 1/1000.

Reference: Royal College of Obstetricians and Gynaecologists (2008). Diagnostic hysteroscopy under general anaesthesia. Consent Advice No. 1. London.

26. Answer: C.

Explanation: Residual stump cancer of the cervix is rare with an incidence of 0.3% and not usually of concern where there is a well-established cervical cytology screening programme in place.

Reference: Shepherd JH, Marcus E (2011). *Shaw's Textbook of Operative Gynaecology*, 7th ed. India: Elsevier.

27. Answer: C.

Explanation: Risk of uterine perforation at the time of surgical evacuation is up to 5 in 1000 women (uncommon).

Reference: Royal College of Obstetricians and Gynaecologists (2010). Surgical evacuation of the uterus for early pregnancy loss. Consent Advice No. 10. London.

28. Answer: B.

Explanation: The risk of ureteric injury at the time of caesarean section is 3 women in every 10,000 (rare).

Reference: Royal College of Obstetricians and Gynaecologists (2009). Caesarean section. Consent Advice No. 7. London.

29. Answer: E.

Explanation: In a review by the Council of the Association of Surgeons it was suggested that, after two failed attempts to insert the Veress needle, either the open (Hasson) technique or Palmer's point entry should be used.

Reference: Royal College of Obstetricians and Gynaecologists (2008). Green-top Guideline No. 49. Preventing entry-related gynaecological laparoscopic injuries. London.

30. Answer: B.

Explanation: If there is concern that the bowel may be adherent under the umbilicus, the primary trocar site should be visualized from a secondary port site, preferably with a 5-mm laparoscope.

Reference: Royal College of Obstetricians and Gynaecologists (2008). Green-top Guideline No. 49. Preventing entry-related gynaecological laparoscopic injuries. London.

31. Answer: C.

Explanation: The type of repair should be selected according to the site and type of injury. In cases of major ureteric injuries (transection and resection) the suggested techniques are site-specific.

- At the upper third of the ureter an end-to-end reanastomosis of the ureter (ureteroureterostomy) should be performed.
- At the middle third either a ureteroureterostomy or a transureteroureterostomy (end-to-side anastomosis of the injured ureter with the contralateral healthy ureter) can be performed.
- At the lower third ureteroneocystostomy (reimplantation of the ureter into the bladder) is preferred. A psoas hitch or a Boari flap

can be performed if a tension-free anastomosis cannot be achieved by simple reimplantation.

Reference: Minas V, Gul N, Aust T, Doyle M, Rowlands D (2014). Urinary tract injuries in laparoscopic gynaecological surgery; prevention, recognition and management. *The Obstetrician & Gynaecologist* 16, 19–28.

32. Answer: A.

Explanation: Management of uterine perforation will depend on the procedure being performed and on the instruments used. If a perforation occurs when using a dilator, hysteroscope (up to 5 mm), curette or during coil insertion, then antibiotics, observation and explanation to the patient is all that is necessary. If larger diameter instruments are used, tissues grasped and avulsion attempted, or if there is significant revealed bleeding from a uterine tear, then laparoscopy should be performed.

Reference: Shakir F, Diab Y (2013). The perforated uterus. *The Obstetrician & Gynaecologist* 15, 256–261.

33. Answer: A.

Explanation: This is likely to be AKI complicated by hyperkalaemia. Immediate treatment of hyperkalaemia is 10 ml 10% calcium gluconate intravenously over 2 to 5 minutes. This stabilizes the myocardium rapidly, but has no effect on serum potassium concentration. The onset of action of calcium gluconate is 2 to 4 minutes and duration of action is 30 to 60 minutes.

Reference: Lobo DN, Lewington AJP, Allison SP (2013). *Basic Concepts of Fluid and Electrolyte Therapy.* Melsungen, Germany: Bibliomed.

Module 7   Surgical procedures

QUESTIONS

34. You are assisting your consultant in a radical hysterectomy and bilateral pelvic lymphadenectomy.

Which of the following instruments will you use to grasp the nodal tissue?

Options

    A. Meigs–Navratil forceps.
    B. DeBakey forceps.
    C. Singley forceps.
    D. Artery forceps.
    E. Kocher forceps.

35. A 29-year-old para 1 undergoes a radical hysterectomy with bilateral pelvic lymphadenectomy for Stage 1B squamous cell carcinoma of the cervix.

Which of the following is not a routine step in this procedure?

Options

    A. Ligation of the uterine vessels close to their source.
    B. Exposure of the ureters to their insertion into the bladder.
    C. Excision of the paracervical tissues.
    D. Oophorectomy.
    E. Excision of the vaginal cuff.

36. Suture materials have different physical properties.

Which of the following is the property by which a suture is capable of supporting acute angulation without breaking or opposing excessive resistance?

Options

    A. Tensile strength.
    B. Elasticity.
    C. Flexibility.
    D. Plasticity.
    E. Handling.

37. Polydioxanone (PDS) is synthetic, absorbable monofilament surgical suture material. It is particularly useful when a combination of an absorbable suture and extended wound support is desirable.

Which of the following best describes the breaking strength retention (tensile strength) of 3-0 PDS at 6 weeks?

Options

    A. 40%.
    B. 50%.
    C. 60%.
    D. 70%.
    E. 80%.

38. You see a 38-year-old para 2 in your gynaecology outpatient clinic who presents with an 8-month history of lower abdominal pain and menorrhagia. A pelvic ultrasound scan shows an enlarged uterus with multiple intramural fibroids, the largest of which is 8 cm in diameter. Her haemoglobin level is 88 g/L. You discuss hysterectomy after a course of GnRH analogue.

Which of the following best describes the effect of GnRH analogue on the volume of the uterine fibroids?

Options

    A. 20% reduction.
    B. 30% reduction.
    C. 40% reduction.
    D. 50% reduction.
    E. 60% reduction.

39. You see a 28-year-old woman with a 2-year history of primary subfertility in your preoperative assessment clinic. She is booked for hysteroscopic resection of a type 1 submucous fibroid, and you obtain her consent for the procedure.

What is the risk of fluid overload associated with operative hysteroscopy?

Options

    A. Around 0.02%.
    B. Around 0.2%.
    C. Around 2%.
    D. Around 12%.
    E. Around 20%.

40. A 64-year-old para 4 is undergoing a vaginal hysterectomy for procidentia. At the end of the anterior vaginal wall closure the vaginal vault could be pulled to the introitus.

What is the most appropriate next step to avoid vaginal vault prolapse?

Options

    A. Suturing the cardinal and uterosacral ligaments to the vaginal cuff.
    B. McCall's culdoplasty.
    C. Colpocleisis.
    D. Prophylactic sacrospinous fixation.
    E. Moschowitz culdoplasty.

41. You are preparing a teaching session to your junior colleagues on the use and safety of electrosurgery in laparoscopy. You discuss the different types of currents produced by the electrosurgical unit (generator).

Which of the following describes the cutting current?

Options

    A. Pulsed waveform, lower frequency, higher voltage.
    B. Pulsed waveform, higher frequency, lower voltage.
    C. Continuous waveform, higher frequency, lower voltage.
    D. Pulsed waveform, higher frequency, higher voltage.
    E. Continuous waveform, lower frequency, higher voltage.

42. You see a 36-year-old woman in your gynaecology clinic. She presents with pelviabdominal mass. Ultrasound scan shows a single, large uterine fibroid. You counsel her regarding management options. She wishes to avoid surgical management and has read about UAE on the Internet.

What is the rate of hysterectomy for women undergoing UAE at 5 years?

Options

    A. 18%.
    B. 28%.
    C. 38%.
    D. 48%.
    E. 58%.

43. You see a 35-year-old para 3 in your outpatient hysteroscopy clinic. She wants to be sterilized and undergoes hysteroscopic sterilization using the Essure device.

What postprocedure advice will you offer her?

Options

    A. Backup contraceptive cover for 3 months.
    B. Backup contraceptive cover for 1 month.
    C. Backup contraceptive cover is unnecessary.
    D. Tubal occlusion should be confirmed in 6 weeks.
    E. Tubal occlusion confirmatory test is unnecessary.

Module 7 Surgical procedures

ANSWERS

34. Answer: C.

Explanation: Singley forceps are used to grasp nodal tissue during pelvic and paraaortic lymph node dissection. They are similar to Russian forceps except that they are lighter and have a central defect. The concentric transverse ridges allow for an improved ability to grasp and place counter traction on lymph nodes.

Reference: Lopes T, Spirtos N, Naik R, Monaghan J (2010). Instruments, operative materials and basic surgical techniques. In: *Bonney's Gynaecological Surgery*, 11th ed. London: Wiley-Blackwell. 15–31.

35. Answer: D.

Explanation: The ovaries do not need to be removed routinely in young women. The incidence of metastases in the ovary is low (1%) in squamous cell carcinoma of the cervix. This must, however, be discussed with each patient individually.

Reference: Acheson N, Luesley D (2010). Cervical cancer standards of care. In: *Gynaecological Oncology for the MRCOG and Beyond*, 2nd ed. London: RCOG Press. 155–167.

36. Answer: C.

Explanation:
- Tensile strength retention is the ability of a thread to oppose traction.
- Elasticity is the capacity of a suture to elongate under traction.
- Flexibility is the property by which a suture is capable of supporting acute angulation without breaking or opposing excessive resistance.
- Plasticity is the lack of recovery of the initial dimensions of the suture after forced lengthening.

- Handling is a property that cannot be measured with instruments but is a special and subjective quality assessed only by the surgeon's hand.

Reference: Mencaglia L, Minelli L, Wattiez A (2013). *Manual of Gynecological Laparoscopic Surgery*, 2nd ed. Tuttlingen, Germany: Endo Press. 74–86.

37. Answer: C.

Explanation: The breaking strength retention (tensile strength of suture in vivo) of 3-0 PDS sutures is 80% at 2 weeks, 70% at 4 weeks and 60% at 6 weeks.

38. Answer: C.

Explanation: Most studies suggest a fibroid volume reduction of 40% with GnRH analogue administration.

Reference: West CP, Lumsden MA, Lawson S, Williamson J, Baird DT (1987). Shrinkage of uterine fibroids during therapy with goserelin (Zoladex): A luteinising hormone-releasing hormone agonist administered as a monthly subcutaneous depot. *Fertility and Sterility* (48) 45–51.

39. Answer: B.

Explanation: The incidence of fluid overload associated with operative hysteroscopy has been estimated to be about 0.1% to 0.2%.

Reference: Munro MG, et al. (2012). AAGL Practice Report: Practice Guidelines for the Management of Hysteroscopic Distending Media. *Journal of Minimally Invasive Gynecology* 20 (2), 137–148.

40. Answer: D.

Explanation: Prophylactic sacrospinous fixation has been suggested at the time of vaginal hysterectomy for marked uterovaginal prolapse when the vault (point C on the POP-Q system) can be pulled as far as the introitus at the end of anterior vaginal wall closure.

Reference: Royal College of Obstetricians and Gynaecologists (2007). Green-top Guideline No 46. The management of post hysterectomy vaginal vault prolapse. London.

41. Answer: C.

Explanation: The electrosurgical unit (generator) produces two general types of current depending on the waveform.

- Cutting current (continuous waveform, higher frequency and lower voltage). It produces rapid and focal tissue heating and cutting effect.
- Coagulation current (pulsed waveform, lower frequency and higher voltage). It produces a lower heat, which causes protein denaturation.

Reference: Feldman L, Fuchshuber P, Jones DB (2012). *The SAGES Manual on the Fundamental Use of Surgical Energy (FUSE)*. New York: Springer-Verlag.

42. Answer: B.

Explanation: An RCT of 177 patients treated by UAE or hysterectomy reported that 28% (23/81) of UAE-treated patients had required hysterectomy at 5-year follow-up.

Reference: National Institute for Clinical Excellence (2010). Uterine artery embolisation for fibroids. National Institute for Health and Care Excellence Interventional Procedures Guidance. London. Available at: https://www.nice.org.uk/guidance/ipg367.

43. Answer: A.

Explanation: The Essure Confirmation Test is a modified HSG used to evaluate the location of the inserts and occlusion of the fallopian tubes. Every patient must have an Essure Confirmation Test 3 months following the Essure placement procedure. The patient must use alternative contraception (except an intrauterine device or intrauterine system) until the test verifies satisfactory location and bilateral occlusion.

Reference: Mitchell S, May J (2014). Correct placement of the Essure device detected by transvaginal ultrasound at one month predicts correct placement at three months. *International Journal of Reproduction, Contraception, Obstetrics and Gynecology* 3 (1), 75–78.

Module 8   Antenatal care

QUESTIONS

44. You are seeing a patient at antenatal clinic at 16 weeks' gestation to make a plan for her antenatal care. The midwife wants to know if the woman has any major risk factors for an SGA fetus.

Which of the following is a major risk factor for this?

Options

    A. BMI of 19.
    B. Chronic hypertension.
    C. PAPP-A > 4 MoM on combined screening.
    D. Preeclampsia in a previous pregnancy.
    E. Smoking 10 cigarettes per day.

45. You see a 34-year-old para 1 with a BMI of 29 in your antenatal clinic. She is at 10 weeks' gestation with a confirmed intrauterine pregnancy and is taking folic acid 400 mcg daily. In her last pregnancy, 3 years ago, she developed preeclampsia at 37 weeks' gestation. She was induced and spontaneously delivered a healthy female at 37^{+2} weighing 2990 g. She has no additional risk factors.

Which of the following would be the best initial antenatal management plan?

Options

    A. Aspirin 75 mg from 18 weeks' gestation until delivery, serial symphysis fundal height at each antenatal visit plotted on a customized growth chart, uterine artery Doppler at 20 to 24 weeks' gestation and, if this is normal, scan for fetal size and UA Doppler in the third trimester.
    B. Aspirin 75 mg from 12 weeks' gestation until delivery and serial symphysis fundal height at each antenatal visit plotted on a customized growth chart.
    C. Aspirin 75 mg from 12 weeks' gestation until delivery, serial symphysis fundal height at each antenatal visit plotted on a customized growth chart, serial ultrasound measurement of fetal

41

size and assessment of fetal well-being with UA Doppler from 26 to 28 weeks' gestation.

D. Aspirin 75 mg from 12 weeks' gestation until delivery, serial symphysis fundal height at each antenatal visit plotted on a customized growth chart, uterine artery Doppler at 20 to 24 weeks' gestation and, if this is normal, scan for fetal size and UA Doppler in third trimester.

E. Aspirin 75 mg from 12 weeks' gestation until 34 weeks' gestation and serial symphysis fundal height at each antenatal visit plotted on a customized growth chart.

46. A 35-year-old para 1 at 32 weeks' gestation is being monitored for an SGA fetus after her midwife plotted symphysis fundal height on a customized growth chart suggested static growth. Her antenatal care has previously been uneventful other than a course of steroids at 26⁺³ weeks' gestation during an admission for threatened preterm labour. Her first delivery was 3 years ago at 39 weeks with the delivery of a healthy male infant weighing 2950 g. She has had tuberculosis as a child living in India, but is otherwise fit and well. Ultrasound scan today reveals the fetal abdominal circumference to be around the 7th centile on a customized chart, with an UA pulsatility index greater than 2 standard deviations from the mean for gestational age. End diastolic flow is present.

What would be the best initial follow-up plan for her?

Options

A. Course of antenatal steroids, daily UA Doppler and weekly abdominal circumference or estimated fetal weight.

B. Course of antenatal steroids, twice weekly UA Doppler and weekly abdominal circumference or estimated fetal weight.

C. Course of antenatal steroids, twice weekly CTG, weekly UA Doppler and weekly abdominal circumference or estimated fetal weight.

D. Twice weekly CTG, weekly UA Doppler and weekly abdominal circumference or estimated fetal weight.

E. Twice weekly UA Doppler with once weekly abdominal circumference or estimated fetal weight.

47. A 25-year-old para 0 with a twin pregnancy has just had a 24-week ultrasound scan at the antenatal clinic. The report shows twin 1 with a DVP of liquor measuring 1.4 cm and twin 2 with a DVP of 10.8 cm. Her 12-week scan report says 'T sign clearly seen'.

What is the most likely diagnosis?

Options

- A. Chromosomal abnormality twin 1.
- B. Cytomegalovirus.
- C. Discordant fetal growth.
- D. Twin reversed arterial perfusion.
- E. Twin-to-twin transfusion syndrome.

48. A 28-year-old para 1 (SVD 3 years ago) who is RhD negative is found to have an anti-D level of 6 IU/ml at a routine 28-week red cell antibody screen. The father is homozygous RhD positive. She is offered weekly ultrasound scans to detect fetal anaemia.

What would be the indication for referral to fetal medicine centre for consideration of intrauterine transfusion?

Options

- A. Ductus venosus Doppler resistance index greater than 1.5 multiples of the median or other signs of fetal anaemia.
- B. Middle cerebral artery Doppler peak systolic velocities greater than 1.5 multiples of the median or other signs of fetal anaemia.
- C. Middle cerebral artery Doppler pulsatility index greater than 1.5 multiples of the median or other signs of fetal anaemia.
- D. Umbilical artery Doppler peak systolic velocities greater than 1.5 multiples of the median or other signs of fetal anaemia.
- E. Umbilical artery Doppler pulsatility index greater than 1.5 multiples of the median or other signs of fetal anaemia.

49. A 19-year-old para 0 is found to have anti-K antibodies at a titre of 8 IU/ml after her 28-week routine antibody screen. She thinks the baby was conceived while on holiday abroad and has no contact with the father.

What is the next step in her management?

Options

- A. Amniocentesis.
- B. Cordocentesis.
- C. Free fetal DNA.
- D. Repeat antibody titre in 2 weeks.
- E. Repeat antibody titre in 4 weeks.

50. A 41-year-old para 2 has multiple fetal anomalies found at a routine 20-week anomaly ultrasound scan. An amniocentesis is performed and trisomy 13 is diagnosed. After counselling, she opts for medical termination of pregnancy, which is performed at 21^{+3} weeks' gestation. She is found to be Rh negative. A Kleihauer test confirms a fetal maternal haemorrhage of 4 ml.

What total dose of anti-D immunoglobulin is required?

Options

- A.   250 IU.
- B.   500 IU.
- C.   625 IU.
- D.   750 IU.
- E.   1000 IU.

51. A 31-year-old para 1 homeless heroin misuser with unknown dates books late and is found to be at approximately 28 weeks' gestation on ultrasound. She is also found to be Rh negative and receives routine antenatal anti-D immunoglobulin (Ig) prophylaxis of 500 IU, with a plan for a further 500 IU at approximately 34 weeks' gestation. One week after her initial anti-D Ig injection, now at around 30 weeks' gestation, she has an episode of a small amount of postcoital spotting. The cervix is healthy and closed, and the placenta is not low.

What is the best management with regards to anti-D?

Options

- A. Anti-D Ig 500 IU now, Kleihauer test, no further routine antenatal anti-D prophylaxis.
- B. Anti-D Ig 500 IU now, Kleihauer test, then routine 500 IU at 34 weeks as planned.
- C. Anti-D Ig 500 IU now, Kleihauer test, then anti-D 500 IU at 35 weeks' gestation.
- D. Kleihauer test now. If fetal maternal haemorrhage less than 4 ml, no anti-D now but routine anti-D Ig at 34 weeks' gestation.
- E. Kleihauer test now. If fetal maternal haemorrhage less than 8 ml, no anti-D now but routine anti-D Ig at 34 weeks.

52. A 32-year-old para 0 is seen for antenatal booking at 10 weeks' gestation. She is a keen outdoor activity enthusiast and asks you about a list of activities she is thinking of doing on her holidays while pregnant.

Which of her planned activities is it most important to strongly advise her against?

Options

- A. Mountain biking.
- B. Open-water swimming.
- C. Scuba diving.
- D. Skiing.
- E. Snorkelling.

53. A 39-year-old para 0 who is 12^{+2} by last menstrual period attends for dating scan. She is keen to have screening for aneuploidy. The CRL is found to be 89 mm.

What would be the best management with regard to dating the pregnancy and screening for Down syndrome?

Options

    A. Date the pregnancy using biparietal diameter and arrange quadruple test for Down syndrome screening.

    B. Date the pregnancy using CRL, measure the nuchal translucency and use the combined test to screen for Down, Edward's and Patau's syndromes.

    C. Date the pregnancy using head circumference and arrange quadruple test for Down syndrome screening.

    D. Date the pregnancy using head circumference, measure nuchal translucency and use the combined test to screen for Down, Edward's and Patau's syndromes.

    E. Date the pregnancy using head circumference, offer amniocentesis to screen for Down, Edward's and Patau's syndromes.

54. A 32-year-old para 0 undergoes IVF outside the UK and has a trichorionic triamniotic triplet pregnancy. She is concerned about how she will cope with her pregnancy towards her due date and asks the latest she is likely to be delivered by.

When should women with trichorionic triamniotic triplets be offered elective delivery, in the absence of prior complications or labour?

Options

    A. From 32^{+0} weeks' gestation, after a course of antenatal corticosteroids.

    B. From 35^{+0} weeks' gestation.

    C. From 35^{+0} weeks' gestation, after a course of antenatal corticosteroids.

    D. From 36^{+0} weeks' gestation, after a course of antenatal corticosteroids.

    E. From 36^{+0} weeks' gestation.

55. You are asked to update a guideline for your unit on antenatal and postnatal care of women suffering from domestic violence.

Approximately what percentage of women receiving antenatal or postnatal care in the UK reports a history of domestic violence?

Options

- A. 5%.
- B. 8%.
- C. 20%.
- D. 35%.
- E. 40%.

56. A 29-year-old primigravida is found to be breech at a 36-week midwife antenatal clinic. This is confirmed on ultrasound scan. She declines ECV and you book a planned caesarean section for 39 weeks' gestation.

What are the chances of the baby spontaneously turning to cephalic?

Options

- A. 5%.
- B. 8%.
- C. 10%.
- D. 12%.
- E. 15%.

57. You see a couple for preconceptual counselling. They are both fit and well with no medical history. The woman's father (now deceased) had haemophilia A.

What are the chances of the couple having a child affected by haemophilia A?

Options

- A. 12.5%.
- B. 25%.
- C. 50%.
- D. 75%.
- E. 100%.

58. A 29-year-old para 0 at 36^{+0} weeks' gestation is referred by a community midwife with a BP of 148/97 mm Hg and 2+ proteinuria at a routine antenatal check. On arrival at hospital her BP is 146/95 mm Hg and repeat is 149/93. The protein : creatinine ratio (PCR) is 37 mg/mmol, but renal function, full blood count, transaminases and bilirubin are normal. The CTG is also normal.

What would be the best initial management plan?

Options

- A. Admit, BP four times per day, ultrasound fetal size, liquor volume and UA Doppler.
- B. Admit, BP four times per day, ultrasound fetal size, liquor volume and UA Doppler and commence antihypertensive treatment.
- C. Admit, BP four times per day, ultrasound fetal size, liquor volume and UA Doppler and commence course of antenatal steroids.
- D. Admit, BP four times per day, ultrasound fetal size, liquor volume and UA Doppler, daily repeat blood tests and urine PCR.
- E. Ultrasound fetal size, liquor volume and UA Doppler, allow home to return in 2 days for CTG and repeat blood tests, BP and urine PCR.

59. You are asked to update your unit guidelines on antenatal aspirin.

Which of the following patients should have aspirin 75 mg daily from 12 weeks' gestation?

Options

- A. 23-year-old primigravida with a BMI of 36 at booking.
- B. 32-year-old para 1 whose mother developed preeclampsia at 27 weeks' gestation.
- C. 34-year-old para 1 with a BMI of 34 at booking who developed gestational diabetes in her previous pregnancy.
- D. 39-year-old para 1 (previous unexplained stillbirth at 36 weeks' gestation).
- E. 39-year-old para 1 (who delivered an SGA baby at 35 weeks, 12 years ago).

60. A 25-year-old primigravida develops severe preeclampsia at 27 weeks' gestation and is delivered by emergency caesarean section. She is concerned about her future pregnancies.

What is the chance of her developing preeclampsia in her next pregnancy?

Options

    A. 16%.
    B. 25%.
    C. 30%.
    D. 40%.
    E. 55%.

61. A 32-year-old nulliparous woman attends for preconception counselling. She had a laparoscopic gastric band procedure 3 months ago.

What is the minimum amount of time pregnancy should be delayed after bariatric surgery?

Options

    A. 6 months.
    B. 9 months.
    C. 12 months.
    D. 18 months.
    E. 24 months.

62. A 32-year-old primigravida at 33^{+6} weeks' gestation has been under close surveillance after a diagnosis of an SGA fetus. She attends for ultrasound in the morning clinic. Fetal abdominal circumference remains less than the 10th centile, DVP of liquor measures 1.2 cm and the UA Doppler shows reversed end diastolic flow. The CTG is normal. A course of antenatal corticosteroids was completed 2 days ago. She had a large breakfast 4 hours ago. The labour ward is busy, an elective caesarean section has just been commenced, but you have access to open an emergency second operating theatre. She is keen for a vaginal delivery.

What would be the best management plan you would advise for her?

Options

- A. Commence induction on the antenatal ward.
- B. Commence induction on the labour ward under close surveillance.
- C. Deliver by caesarean section today.
- D. Deliver by category 1 caesarean section.
- E. Repeat ultrasound and umbilical Doppler twice weekly, aiming to deliver at 37 weeks.

63. A primigravida at 20 weeks' gestation attends obstetric triage feeling short of breath. She has a monochorionic diamniotic twin pregnancy. She has not attended for antenatal care since her dating scan at 14 weeks' gestation where chorionicity was confirmed, after which she separated from her partner. Chest examination is unremarkable, but her SFH is 32 cm.

An ultrasound scan is performed, revealing that both twins are alive. Twin 1 has polyhydramnios with a DVP of liquor measuring 9.5 cm and bladder visible. Twin 2 has oligohydramnios with a DVP of liquor measuring 0.5 cm. Despite an hour of scanning, it is not possible to identify a bladder in twin 2. Both twins have end diastolic flow present on UA Doppler. A diagnosis of suspect twin–twin transfusion syndrome is made.

What Quintero stage would this be classified as?

Options

    A. I.
    B. II.
    C. III.
    D. IV.
    E. V.

64. A 28-year-old primigravida with monochorionic diamniotic twins comes for her regular ultrasound and antenatal clinic appointment at 24 weeks. Twin 2 has no fetal heart present and Spalding's sign is present. Twin 1 has a fundal height with normal size, liquor volume, UA Doppler and a visible bladder with plenty of fetal movement. An ultrasound 2 weeks ago had been normal. Her BP is normal and there is no proteinuria.

After a single fetal death in a monochorionic diamniotic twin pregnancy, what is the overall rate of survival for the co-twin?

Options

    A. 68%.
    B. 72%.
    C. 88%.
    D. 93%.
    E. 97%.

Module 8 Antenatal care

ANSWERS

44. Answer: B.

Explanation: A major risk factor for SGA neonates is defined as an odds ratio of greater than 2.0. A BMI of 19, smoking 10 cigarettes per day and preeclampsia in a previous pregnancy are all minor risk factors. PAPP-A (pregnancy-associated plasma protein-A) is a protein checked for on blood test at the combined aneuploid screen. A low PAPP-A < 0.4 MoM (multiples of median) at combined screening is a major risk factor, not a raised PAPP-A.

Reference: Royal College of Obstetricians and Gynaecologists (2013). Green-top Guideline No. 31, Small for gestational age, 2nd ed. London.

45. Answer: B.

Explanation: Previous preeclampsia is a minor risk factor for an SGA neonate. In the absence of any other risk factors, no additional ultrasound scanning is needed unless other risk factors develop, or a symphysis fundal height (SFH) measurement is less than the 10th centile, or there is reduced SFH growth velocity. Previous preeclampsia is, however, considered a major risk factor for recurrent preeclampsia, and aspirin should be taken from 12 weeks' gestation to delivery.

Reference: National Institute for Health and Care Excellence (2010). Clinical guideline 107. Hypertension in pregnancy. Royal College of Obstetricians and Gynaecologists Green-top Guideline No. 31. Small for gestational age, 2nd ed. London.

46. Answer: E.

Explanation: A single course of antenatal steroids should be given to pregnancies affected by fetal growth restriction at 24^{+0} to 35^{+6} weeks' gestation at risk of delivery. A second 'rescue' course may be considered with senior input if the first course was given before 26^{+0}; this woman should, therefore, not have further antenatal steroids. The management would be twice-weekly Doppler. CTG should not be used alone. Weekly abdominal circumference (AC) or estimated fetal weight (EFW) is recommended to assess size, although this should not be used to assess growth unless the measurements are at least 3 weeks apart.

References: Royal College of Obstetrics and Gynaecologists (2013). Green-top Guideline No. 31. Small for gestational age, 2nd ed. London.
Royal College of Obstetricians and Gynaecologists (2010). Green-top Guideline No. 7. Antenatal corticosteroids to reduce neonatal morbidity and mortality, 4th ed. London.

47. Answer: E.

Explanation: A T sign at a 12-week scan is strongly correlated with a monochorionic pregnancy, the majority of which are monochorionic-diamniotic. Twin 1 has oligohydramnios and twin 2 has polyhydramnios. While discordant fetal growth is possible, twin-to-twin transfusion syndrome is more likely.

Reference: Royal College of Obstetricians and Gynaecologists (2008). Green-top Guideline No. 51. Monochorionic twin pregnancy management. London.

48. Answer: B.

Explanation: It is the MCA Doppler peak systolic velocity. The pulsatility index may, in some situations, be used as part of the assessment for an SGA fetus, but not for monitoring for fetal anaemia. The others are not useful. Should this threshold be met, the fetus would be considered for intrauterine transfusion or, at later gestations, delivery.

Reference: Royal College of Obstetricians and Gynaecologists (2014). Green-top Guideline No. 65. The management of women with red cell antibodies during pregnancy. London.

49. Answer: C.

Explanation: Anti-K titres correlate poorly with the severity of the disease; fetal anaemia can occur with titres as low as 8 IU/ml. As soon as anti-K is detected, an at-risk fetus needs to be monitored for fetal anaemia. We do not know if this fetus is at risk, however, and, because it is not possible to test the father, the next step must be to check free fetal

DNA from the maternal plasma. If this shows the fetus is K positive, then weekly MCA peak systolic velocities and two-weekly antibody titres should be checked.

Reference: Royal College of Obstetricians and Gynaecologists (2014). Green-top Guideline No. 65. The management of women with red cell antibodies during pregnancy. London.

50. Answer: B.

Explanation: 500 IU anti-D Ig is required for a potentially sensitizing antenatal event after 20 weeks' gestation where fetomaternal haemorrhage is less than or equal to 4 ml.

Reference: Qureshi H, et al. (2014). BCSH guideline for the use of anti-D immunoglobulin for the prevention of haemolytic disease of the fetus and newborn. *Transfusion Medicine* 24 (1), 8–20.

51. Answer: B.

Explanation: Routine antenatal anti-D immunoglobulin prophylaxis (RAADP) should be regarded as supplementary to any anti-D immunoglobulin administered for a potentially sensitizing event. RAADP may be either two doses of 500 IU at 28 and 34 weeks' gestation or one dose of 1500 IU at 28 to 30 weeks' gestation. Given this additional potentially sensitizing antenatal event, further anti-D is required.

Reference: Qureshi H, et al. (2014). BCSH guideline for the use of anti-D immunoglobulin for the prevention of haemolytic disease of the fetus and newborn. *Transfusion Medicine* 24 (1), 8–20.

52. Answer: C.

Explanation: While the others may present some hazards, scuba diving and the risk of fetal decompression sickness is the most important to avoid.

Reference: National Institute for Health and Care Excellence (2008). Clinical guideline 62. Antenatal care 2008 (modified 2014). London.

53. Answer: C.

Explanation: If the CRL is greater than 84 mm, then the gestation is greater than 14^{+1} weeks and an head circumference should be used to date the pregnancy; the quadruple test (biochemical, not measurement of nuchal translucency) should be performed if screening is desired. Amniocentesis is a diagnostic test, not a screening test.

Reference: National Institute for Health and Care Excellence (2008). Clinical guideline 62. Antenatal care 2008 (modified 2014), NHS Fetal anomaly screening programme 2015–2016. London.

54. Answer C.

Explanation: Women with trichorionic triamniotic triplets should be offered elective delivery in the absence of prior complications or labour from 35^{+0} weeks' gestation, after a course of antenatal corticosteroids.

Reference: National Institute for Health and Care Excellence (2011). Clinical guideline 129. Multiple pregnancies. London.

55. Answer C.

Explanation: About 13% to 24% of women receiving antenatal or postnatal care in the UK report a history of domestic violence.

Reference: Gottlieb A (2012). Domestic violence: A clinical guide for women's healthcare providers. *The Obstetrician & Gynaecologist* 14 (3), 197–202.

56. Answer: B.

Reference: Royal College of Obstetricians and Gynaecologists (2006). Green-top guideline No. 20a. External cephalic version to reduce the incidence of breech presentation. London.

57. Answer: B.

Explanation: Haemophilia A is an X-linked recessive condition. The woman will be an obligate carrier of haemophilia A as she will have received an X chromosome from her father. There is a 25% chance of their child being an affected male, 25% of being a carrier female and 50% chance of them having a child who is neither affected nor a carrier.

Reference: Royal College of Obstetricians and Gynaecologists. StratOG, core training, antenatal care, genetic disorders. https://stratog.rcog.org.uk/. Accessed March 2015.

58. Answer: A.

Explanation: This woman has mild preeclampsia. She should, therefore, be admitted but does not need antihypertensive treatment. Once preeclampsia is diagnosed, her urine protein:creatinine ratio (PCR) should not be repeated. Antenatal corticosteroids are not indicated at this gestation unless elective caesarean section before 39 weeks' gestation is planned.

References: National Institute for Health and Care Excellence (2010). Clinical guideline 107. Hypertension in pregnancy. London.
Royal College of Obstetricians and Gynaecologists (2010). Green-top Guideline No. 7. Antenatal corticosteroids to reduced neonatal morbidity and mortality, 4th ed. London.

59. Answer: A.

Explanation: Those with one major or two or more moderate risk factors for preeclampsia should have aspirin 75 mg per day from 12 weeks' gestation until delivery. First pregnancy and a BMI greater than 35 at first visit are both moderate risk factors.

Reference: National Institute for Health and Care Excellence (2010). Clinical guideline 107. Hypertension in pregnancy. London.

60. Answer: E.

If a woman develops severe preeclampsia, eclampsia, or HELLP syndrome, and needs to be delivered before 28 weeks, then the risk of a future pregnancy being complicated by preeclampsia is 55%.

Reference: National Institute for Health and Care Excellence (2010). Clinical guideline 107. Hypertension in pregnancy. London.

61. Answer: C.

Explanation: The current recommendation is to delay for at least 12 months, as this is the period when rapid weight loss occurs and when nutritional and electrolyte imbalances are more likely to arise. This would theoretically be the time of greatest risk for an adverse perinatal outcome if conception were to occur. There are, however, no substantial clinical data behind this advice.

Reference: Khan R, Dawlatly B, Chappatte O (2013). Pregnancy outcome following bariatric surgery. *The Obstetrician & Gynaecologist* 15 (1) 37–43.

62. Answer: C.

Explanation: With reversed end diastolic flow on UA Doppler at this gestation, delivery is needed by caesarean section. Any attempt at induction of labour is highly likely to result in fetal compromise, because the fetal reserves are likely to be already low. With a normal CTG it would be reasonable to wait a few hours until she is fasted and the first theatre is free – there is no need for a category 1 caesarean section.

Reference: Royal College of Obstetricians and Gynaecologists (2013). Green-top Guideline No. 31. Small for gestational age, 2nd ed. London.

63. Answer: B.

Explanation: The Quintero staging system (from I to V) is used to classify the severity of twin–twin transfusion system (V being the most severe), based on ultrasound findings. In addition to the oligohydramnios/polyhydramnios sequence in this case, it is not possible to identify the bladder in the donor twin, making this Stage II. Critically abnormal Dopplers would be required for Stage III.

Reference: Royal College of Obstetricians and Gynaecologists (2008). Green-top Guideline No. 51. Monochorionic twin pregnancy management. London.

64. Answer: C.

Explanation: Unlike with dichorionic twins, death of a monochorionic twin results in hazardous acute haemodynamic changes in the co-twin.

By the time of diagnosis of the death, the damage to the co-twin will have probably already occurred. The overall risk of death to the co-twin is 12%, with an additional 18% chance of neurologic disability.

Reference: Royal College of Obstetricians and Gynaecologists (2008). Green-top Guideline No. 51. Monochorionic twin pregnancy management. London.

QUESTIONS

65. You are asked to see a 28-year-old woman who is day 2 following a caesarean section for unsuccessful induction of labour at 37 weeks' gestation. She was diagnosed with mild preeclampsia at 36 weeks' gestation. Her blood pressure has been 155/100 mm Hg on two occasions today, although she is asymptomatic and her deep tendon reflexes are normal. She is breast feeding. You decide to start her on an antihypertensive agent.

Which of the following antihypertensive agents has insufficient evidence on infant safety to recommend for use in breast feeding mothers?

Options

    A. Amlodipine.
    B. Atenolol.
    C. Captopril.
    D. Enalapril.
    E. Metoprolol.

66. You have been asked to see a 37-year-old para 1 at 25 weeks' gestation. She had an elective caesarean section for breech presentation at 39 weeks in her first pregnancy. This is her second pregnancy, and she now describes a small painless lump in her right breast, which she has discovered accidentally. There is no history of bleeding per nipple. She is worried as she has a strong family history of breast cancer and you arrange an urgent referral to the specialist breast team.

What is the most appropriate first-line imaging modality?

Options

    A. Gadolinium-enhanced magnetic resonance imaging.
    B. Mammography with fetal shielding.
    C. Ultrasound-guided aspiration for cytology.
    D. Ultrasound-guided biopsy for histology.
    E. Ultrasound scan.

67. A 33-year-old asylum seeker from Somalia is referred by the community midwife to the antenatal clinic, and you see her with an interpreter. She is 22 weeks into her first ongoing pregnancy and reports that she was subjected to female genital cutting when she turned 12 years of age. She also gives a history of recurrent urinary tract infections. Examination of the vulva shows that the clitoris, labia minora and labia majora are surgically removed.

Which of the following female genital mutilation types describe these findings?

Options

    A. I.
    B. II.
    C. III.
    D. IV.
    E. V

68. You see a 31-year-old primigravida at 26 weeks' gestation who presents with worsening fatigue, sweating, insomnia, loss of weight and palpitations. She reports good fetal movements. Physical examination shows exophthalmos, an enlarged nontender thyroid gland and fine hand tremors. Her thyroid function test results show a TSH less than 0.05 mU/L (normal range 0.4–5.0) and a T_4 of 70 pmol/L (normal range 10–20). You counsel her regarding the risks of poorly controlled hyperthyroidism in pregnancy.

Which of the following is not a recognized risk?

Options

    A. Stillbirth.
    B. Intrauterine growth restriction.
    C. Preeclampsia.
    D. Congestive cardiac failure.
    E. Gestational diabetes.

69. You are asked to see a woman on the postnatal ward. She sustained a grade 3B perineal tear following an instrumental delivery. The tear was appropriately repaired with an overlapping technique using 3-0 PDS suture in theatre.

What advice would you give her regarding the prognosis following surgical repair?

Options

- A. 60% of women are asymptomatic at 12 months.
- B. 55% of women are asymptomatic at 12 months.
- C. 50% of women are asymptomatic at 12 months.
- D. 45% of women are asymptomatic at 12 months.
- E. 40% of women are asymptomatic at 12 months.

70. You see a 22-year-old para 1 who is 35 weeks into her second pregnancy. She presents to the labour ward complaining of headache, abdominal pain, nausea, vomiting and widespread itching with no rash. On examination there is mild jaundice and bilateral lower limb oedema. Her BP is 150/95 mm Hg, and urinalysis shows 1+ protein. Your differential diagnosis includes preeclampsia, HELLP (haemolysis, elevated liver enzymes, and low platelet count) syndrome, acute fatty liver of pregnancy (AFLP) and haemolytic uraemic syndrome. You request FBC, LFT, U&E, clotting screen and serum urate.

What is the single most important test that could help to distinguish AFLP from the other potential problems?

Options

- A. Blood film.
- B. Creatinine.
- C. Glucose.
- D. Lactate dehydrogenase.
- E. Urine protein : creatinine ratio.

71. You see a 31-year-old primigravida at 37 weeks who presents to your day assessment unit with headache and blurring of vision. Her BP is 160/110 mm Hg, and urine dipstick shows 3+ protein. Her reflexes are brisk with four beats of ankle clonus, and her abdomen is soft. The symphysis fundal height is 35 cm, the CTG is normal and her urine protein : creatinine ratio is 90 mg/mmol.

What is the most appropriate action?

Options

- A. Fluid restriction to 125 ml/h with magnesium sulphate infusion followed by delivery of the baby.
- B. Fluid restriction to 125 ml/h with magnesium sulphate infusion followed by hydralazine and delivery of the baby.
- C. Fluid restriction to 80 ml/h with magnesium sulphate infusion followed by hydralazine and delivery of the baby.
- D. Magnesium sulphate infusion followed by hydralazine and delivery of the baby.
- E. Immediate delivery of the baby.

72. You see a 23-year-old woman, who is known to have beta thalassaemia major. She underwent splenectomy at the age of 7. Her platelet count is 660×10^9/L at booking.

What antenatal thromboprophylaxis is recommended?

Options

- A. Low-dose aspirin 75 mg/day.
- B. LMWH.
- C. Low-dose aspirin 75 mg/day and LMWH.
- D. LMWH for 6 weeks postnatally.
- E. UFH.

73. A 35-year-old para 1 who is 34 weeks presents to your day assessment unit complaining of pruritus, especially in the palms and soles. She reports good fetal movements and her pregnancy has been uneventful so far. She also gives a history of induction of labour at 38 weeks for obstetric cholestasis in her first pregnancy. Inspection of the skin shows scratch marks but no rash. The SFH is 36 cm and a CTG is normal. Her liver function tests show an elevated alanine transaminase and bile acids. You suspect obstetric cholestasis.

How would you counsel her regarding obstetric cholestasis?

Options

- A. Recurrence rate is 35%.
- B. Postpartum haemorrhage rate is around 35%.
- C. Risk of spontaneous prematurity is around 35%.
- D. Ursodeoxycholic acid improves itching and reduces the incidence of abnormal umbilical artery Doppler studies.
- E. Early term delivery is not associated with increased incidence of caesarean section.

74. You see a 30-year-old para 1 in the antenatal clinic. She is found to have a platelet count of 85×10^9/L on routine screening at 28 weeks' gestation. This is her second pregnancy; her first child was delivered at term by caesarean section for breech presentation. She reports good fetal movements and has no history of bruising or bleeding.

Which of the following conditions could not explain her thrombocytopenia?

Options

- A. Alloimmune thrombocytopenia.
- B. Gestational thrombocytopenia.
- C. Immune thrombocytopenic purpura.
- D. Preeclampsia.
- E. Antiphospholipid syndrome.

75. Normal pregnancy is associated with changes in the cardiovascular system including change in the position of the heart. This results in changes in the ECG.

Which of the following is not a normal ECG finding during pregnancy?

Options

    A. Atrial and ventricular ectopics.

    B. Q-wave (small) and inverted T-wave in lead III.

    C. ST segment depression and T-wave inversion in inferior and lateral leads.

    D. QRS axis leftward shift.

    E. ST segment elevation and T-wave inversion in inferior and lateral leads.

76. You see a 26-year-old para 1 in your day assessment unit. She is at 30 weeks' gestation and presents with sudden onset of fever, malaise and jaundice. She reports recent travel to Kenya. Her observations are temperature 38°C, BP 110/70 mm Hg, pulse rate 90 bpm and respiratory rate 16 per minute. You suspect malaria in pregnancy and arrange a rapid diagnostic test and blood film for malaria parasites. The blood film shows trophozoites of *Plasmodium falciparum* and *P. vivax*. There are no neurologic symptoms or signs, and the electrolytes are normal.

What is your antimalarial agent of choice?

Options

    A. Artesunate.

    B. Quinine and clindamycin.

    C. Chloroquine.

    D. Primaquine.

    E. Primaquine and clindamycin.

77. The midwife on the postnatal ward asks you to make a thromboprophylaxis plan for a 21-year-old woman with sickle cell disease. She is day 1 postnatal following an elective caesarean section for intrauterine growth restriction and has no other risk factors.

Which of the following is the correct plan?

Options

    A. LMWH while in hospital.

    B. LMWH while in hospital and 7 days post-discharge.

    C. LMWH while in hospital and 6 weeks post-discharge.

    D. UFH while in hospital.

    E. UFH while in hospital and for 7 days post-discharge.

78. You see a 30-year-old who is at 17 weeks in her third pregnancy and who presents with a threatened miscarriage. Her blood group is A Rhesus negative. She had surgical management of miscarriage in her second pregnancy and anti-D immunoglobulin was not given. Screening for red cell antibodies shows an anti-D antibodies level of 7 IU/ml. The bleeding has now settled, the pregnancy is ongoing and she is pain free.

What is your most appropriate next step?

Options

    A. Referral to fetal medicine unit.

    B. Repeat anti-D level in 4 weeks.

    C. Repeat anti-D level in 2 weeks.

    D. Offer anti-D immunoglobulin.

    E. Kleihauer–Betke test.

79. You see a 28 year old in your antenatal clinic. She is 17 weeks into her third ongoing pregnancy. Her first pregnancy ended in a spontaneous miscarriage at 13 weeks and, in her second pregnancy, she gave birth to an anaemic baby who required exchange transfusion. Anti-E antibodies were detected at her initial screening in this pregnancy.

What is your most appropriate next step?

Options

- A. Noninvasive fetal genotyping using maternal blood.
- B. Determine paternal E antigen status.
- C. Obtain maternal anti-E level.
- D. Obtain fetal haemoglobin level by cordocentesis.
- E. Monitor fetal middle cerebral artery peak systolic velocity.

80. You see a 36-year-old woman with a BMI of 38 kg/m^2 in your day assessment unit. She is 32 weeks into her fourth ongoing pregnancy and describes sudden onset shortness of breath with no cough or chest pain. She does, however, have right leg pain and swelling. Physical examination shows a pulse rate of 100 bpm, BP 110/70 mm Hg, temperature 37°C and respiratory rate 18 per minute. Chest auscultation is unremarkable. You suspect PE and start LMWH.

What is your next most appropriate test?

Options

- A. CTPA.
- B. Ventilation/perfusion lung scan.
- C. Arterial blood gases.
- D. ECG and chest x-ray.
- E. Compression duplex ultrasound leg studies.

81. You see a 34-year-old primigravida at 32 weeks' gestation in your day assessment unit. She presents with a 2-day history of nonspecific headaches, nausea, retrobulbar pain and blurring of vision. Although a neurologic examination is normal, an ophthalmologic examination shows bilateral papilledema. A magnetic resonance venogram demonstrates no mass lesion or venous thrombosis. A lumbar puncture, however, shows a raised opening pressure (greater than 250 mm H_2O) but with no other cytologic or chemical abnormalities. Her BMI is 36 kg/m^2.

Which of the following is the drug of choice?

Options

    A. Triptan.
    B. Nifedipine.
    C. Labetalol.
    D. Acetazolamide.
    E. Hydrochlorothiazide.

82. You see a 33-year-old woman in the postnatal ward. She was diagnosed with gestational diabetes this pregnancy, and her capillary blood glucose level is 4 mmol/L.

What is her risk of developing type 2 diabetes within 5 years of this birth?

Options

    A. 15%.
    B. 20%.
    C. 30%.
    D. 40%.
    E. 50%.

83. You see a 22-year-old para 0 with systemic lupus erythematosus for preconception counselling. She has had no flares for the last 12 months. Her antibodies screen is negative for anti-Ro/La antibodies, and there is no concurrent antiphospholipid syndrome. She is keen to be pregnant and asks you about the safety of immunosuppressant drugs during pregnancy.

Which of the following drugs does not cross the placenta?

Options

- A. Azathioprine.
- B. Methotrexate.
- C. Mycophenolate mofetil.
- D. Cyclophosphamide.
- E. Ciclosporin.

84. You see a 30-year-old para 3 at 31 weeks' gestation in your day assessment unit. She presents with skin rash and itching. On examination, there are erythematous papules and vesicles all over the abdomen including the umbilicus, limbs, palms and soles.

What is the most likely diagnosis?

Options

- A. Atopic eruption of pregnancy.
- B. Pemphigoid gestationis.
- C. Polymorphic eruption of pregnancy.
- D. Erythema nodosum.
- E. Pityriasis rosea.

Module 9   Maternal medicine

ANSWERS

65. Answer: A.

Explanation: Atenolol, captopril, enalapril and metoprolol are antihypertensive agents with no known adverse effects on infants receiving breast milk.

Reference: Smith M, Waugh J, Nelson-Piercy C (2013). Management of postpartum hypertension. *The Obstetrician & Gynaecologist* 15, 45–50.

66. Answer: E.

Explanation: Ultrasound is used first to assess the lump. Mammography is necessary after cancer is confirmed to assess the extent of disease and the contralateral breast. Cytology is often inconclusive in pregnancy as a result of proliferative changes.

Reference: Royal College of Obstetricians and Gynaecologists (2011). Green-top Guideline No. 12. Pregnancy and breast cancer. London.

67. Answer: B.

Explanation:
   I.   Partial or total removal of the clitoris and/or the prepuce (clitoridectomy).
   II. Partial or total removal of the clitoris and the labia minora, with or without excision of the labia majora (excision).
   III. Narrowing of the vaginal orifice with creation of a covering seal by cutting and appositioning the labia minora and/or the labia majora, with or without excision of the clitoris (infibulation).
   IV. All other harmful procedures to the female genitalia for nonmedical purposes, e.g. pricking, piercing, incising, scraping and cauterizing.

Reference: Royal College of Obstetricians and Gynaecologists (2009). Green-top Guideline No. 53. Female genital mutilation and its management. London.

68. Answer: E.

Explanation: Hypothyroidism is associated with gestational diabetes.

Reference: Collins S, Arulkumaran S, Hayes K, Jackson S, Impey L, Eds. (2013). *Oxford Handbook of Obstetrics and Gynaecology*, 3rd ed., Oxford Medical Handbooks. Oxford, UK: Oxford University Press, 2013.

69. Answer: A.

Explanation: Women should be advised that the prognosis following external anal sphincter (EAS) repair is good, with 60% to 80% asymptomatic at 12 months.

Reference: Royal College of Obstetricians and Gynaecologists (2015). Green-top Guideline No. 29, p. 29. The management of third and fourth degree perineal tears. London.

70. Answer: C.

Explanation: One of the keys to the diagnosis of acute fatty liver of pregnancy is the rapidity with which liver function tests (LFT) can deteriorate in the aggressive phase of the disease. This typically is combined with features of hepatic synthetic failure, including hypoglycaemia, deranged clotting and confusion secondary to hepatic encephalopathy.

Reference: James D, Steer PJ, Weiner CP, Gonik B, Crowther C, Robson S, Eds. (2011). *High Risk Pregnancy:Management Options*, 4th ed. St Louis: Saunders.

71. Answer: C.

Explanation: In women with severe preeclampsia, maintenance fluids should be limited to 80 ml/h unless there are other ongoing fluid losses (e.g. haemorrhage). The BP should be below 150/80 to 100 mm Hg, and consideration should be given to intravenous magnesium sulphate in a woman with severe preeclampsia if birth is planned within 24 hours.

Reference: National Institute for Health and Care Excellence (2010). Clinical guideline 107. Hypertension in pregnancy: The management of hypertensive disorders during pregnancy. London.

72. Answer: C.

Explanation: Women with thalassaemia who have undergone splenectomy and have a platelet count greater than 600×10^9/L should be offered LMWH thromboprophylaxis as well as low-dose aspirin (75 mg/day).

Reference: Royal College of Obstetricians and Gynaecologists (2014). Green-top Guideline No. 66. Management of beta thalassaemia in pregnancy. London.

73. Answer: E.

Explanation: Early term delivery is not associated with increased incidence of caesarean section. Recurrence rate of obstetric cholestasis is 45% to 90%. The risk of postpartum haemorrhage rate is around 22%. The risk of spontaneous prematurity is around 4% to 12%.

References: Royal College of Obstetricians and Gynaecologists (2011). Green-top Guideline No. 43. Obstetric cholestasis. London.

Chappell LC, Gurung V, Seed PT, Chambers J, Williamson C, Thornton JG, et al. (2012). Ursodeoxycholic acid versus placebo, and early term delivery versus expectant management, in women with intrahepatic cholestasis of pregnancy: Semifactorial randomised clinical trial. *BMJ* 344, e3799.

74. Answer: A.

Explanation: Alloimmune thrombocytopenia is a cause of fetal, not maternal, thrombocytopenia. The maternal platelet count is normal in this condition.

Reference: Nelson-Piercy C, Girling J (2007). *Obstetric Medicine*. London: Springer.

75. Answer: E.

Atrial and ventricular ectopics, Q-wave and inverted T-wave in lead III, ST segment depression and T-wave inversion in inferior and lateral leads, and QRS axis leftward shift are ECG changes which can be found in normal pregnancy.

Reference: Nelson-Piercy C (2010). *Handbook of Obstetric Medicine*, 4th ed. Boca Raton, FL: CRC Press.

76. Answer: B.

Explanation: Intravenous artesunate is the treatment of choice for severe falciparum malaria. Quinine and clindamycin are used to treat uncomplicated *Plasmodium falciparum* or mixed, such as *P. falciparum* and *P. vivax*. Chloroquine is used to treat *P. vivax*, *P. ovale* and *P. malariae*. Primaquine should not be used in pregnancy.

Reference: Royal College of Obstetricians and Gynaecologists (2010). Green-top Guideline No. 54b. The diagnosis and treatment of malaria in pregnancy. London.

77. Answer: C.

Explanation: LMWH should be administered while in hospital and 7 days post-discharge following vaginal delivery or for a period of 6 weeks following caesarean section.

Reference: Royal College of Obstetricians and Gynaecologists (2011). Green-top Guideline No. 61. Management of sickle cell disease in pregnancy. London.

78. Answer: A.

Explanation: An anti-D level of between 4 and 15 IU/ml correlates with a moderate risk of haemolytic disease of the fetus and newborn (HDFN). Referral for a fetal medicine opinion should therefore be made when anti-D levels are greater than 4 IU/ml.

Reference: Royal College of Obstetricians and Gynaecologists (2014). The management of women with red cell antibodies during pregnancy. Green-top Guideline No. 65. London.

79. Answer: A.

Explanation: Noninvasive fetal genotyping using maternal blood is now possible for D, C, c, E, e and K antigens. This should be performed for the relevant antigen in the first instance when maternal red cell antibodies are present.

Reference: Royal College of Obstetricians and Gynaecologists (2014). Green-top Guideline No. 65. The management of women with red cell antibodies during pregnancy. London.

80. Answer: E.

Explanation: In women with suspected PE who also have symptoms and signs of deep venous thrombosis (DVT), compression duplex ultrasound should be performed. If compression ultrasonography confirms the presence of DVT, no further investigation is necessary and treatment for venous thromboembolism should continue.

Reference: Royal College of Obstetricians and Gynaecologists (2015). Green-top Guideline No. 37b. Thromboembolic disease in pregnancy and the puerperium: Acute management. London.

81. Answer: D.

Explanation: The most likely diagnosis is idiopathic intracranial hypertension, and acetazolamide is the drug of choice. It inhibits carbonic anhydrase enzyme in the central nervous system, which delays abnormal and excessive discharge of cerebrospinal fluid from the choroid plexus. It is a Category C drug (potential benefits may warrant use of the drug in pregnant women despite potential risks).

Reference: Thirumalaikumar L, Ramalingam K (2014). Idiopathic intracranial hypertension in pregnancy. *The Obstetrician &Gynaecologist* 16, 93–97.

82. Answer: E.

Explanation: Gestational diabetes is one of the strongest risk factors for the subsequent development of type 2 diabetes: up to 50% of women diagnosed with gestational diabetes develop type 2 diabetes within 5 years of the birth.

Reference: National Institute for Health and Care Excellence (2015). Diabetes in pregnancy: Management of diabetes and its complications from preconception to the postnatal period. London.

83. Answer: B.

Explanation: Methotrexate apparently does not cross the placenta, although it has been associated with neural tube defects if used in early pregnancy. It should ideally be stopped before conception.

Reference: Cauldwell M, Nelson-Piercy C (2012). Maternal and fetal complications of systemic lupus erythematosus. *The Obstetrician & Gynaecologist* 14, 167–174.

84. Answer: B.

Explanation: Pemphigoid gestationis is a rare but serious condition. It can occur at any time during pregnancy but usually in the third trimester. Lesions begin in the periumbilical region spreading to limbs, palms and soles. This is unlike polymorphic eruption of pregnancy where the umbilicus is usually spared.

Reference: Nelson-Piercy, C (2010). Skin disease. In: *Handbook of Obstetric Medicine*. Boca Raton, FL: CRC Press, 231–238.

Module 10 Management of labour

85. A 35-year-old para 3 (previous SVDs) at 39 weeks' gestation presents with no fetal movements, and a diagnosis of IUFD is made. She is given mifepristone and then returns 2 days later for misoprostol to induce labour. Repeated doses are given until contractions commence. Contractions develop quickly but she then reports severe continuous pain. On assessment she is profoundly shocked with a tender abdomen and profuse vaginal bleeding. She is taken to theatre and a laparotomy is performed. The abdomen has 4 L of blood, and the uterus is extensively ruptured. Hysterectomy and extensive resuscitation efforts are performed, but unfortunately the woman dies. An inquiry is held and the dose of misoprostol used is criticized for being too high.

What would have been a suitable misoprostol regime to induce labour in this woman?

Options

   A. Misoprostol 25 to 50 mcg 4 hourly.
   B. Misoprostol 200 mcg 4 hourly, then 100 mcg 4 hourly.
   C. Misoprostol 200 mcg 4 hourly.
   D. Misoprostol 200 mcg 4 hourly, followed by misoprostol 25 to 50 mcg 4 hourly.
   E. Misoprostol 400 mcg 4 hourly, followed by misoprostol 25 to 50 mcg 4 hourly.

86. A 39-year-old primigravida presents at 35 weeks' gestation with a 48-hour history of absent fetal movement. An IUFD is diagnosed on ultrasound scan. She is otherwise fit and well and antenatal care has been unremarkable until this point. Labour is induced and a macerated stillborn male weighing 2534 g is delivered. The couple consent to postmortem.

Which of the following would be part of the initial investigations?

Options

- A. Maternal serum for maternal alloimmune antiplatelet antibodies.
- B. Maternal serum for anti-Ro and anti-La antibodies.
- C. Maternal serum thyroid-stimulating hormone, free T_3 and free T_4.
- D. Maternal urine for cocaine metabolites.
- E. Maternal serum for carbon monoxide levels.

87. After a period of training, an obstetric unit introduces STAN for intrapartum fetal monitoring to the labour ward.

Which of the following has STAN been shown to reduce?

Options

- A. Caesarean section rate.
- B. Fetal blood sample rate.
- C. Number of babies born with low Apgar scores at 5 minutes.
- D. Number of babies born with neonatal encephalopathy.
- E. Rate of mental retardation in children at 5 years of age.

88. A 29-year-old para 0 at 40^{+4} weeks' gestation presents to the labour ward with pyrexia, malaise and shortness of breath. While transferring onto her labour room bed, she collapses. She is not breathing and there is no pulse. Cardiopulmonary resuscitation (CPR) is commenced and an emergency call is made. The anaesthetist and his operating department practitioner arrive.

What would be the best airway protection during CPR in this patient?

Options

- A. Intubation with a cuffed endotracheal tube.
- B. Laryngeal mask airway.
- C. Oropharyngeal airway.
- D. Surgical cricothyroidotomy.
- E. Tracheotomy.

89. A 29-year-old para 0 spontaneously labours at 38^{+3} weeks' gestation and at 16:00 she is 5 cm dilated. At 18:00 decelerations are heard on intermittent auscultation and a CTG is commenced. Contractions are 4:10, base rate is 150 bpm variability greater than 5 bpm, there are no accelerations and there are declarations with every contraction, mostly of greater than 60 bpm and often for greater than 60 seconds. On examination at 18:30 the cervix is 9 cm dilated, and the fetus is direct occiput anterior at spines. A decision is made for fetal blood sampling. Three good samples are taken at 18:40, and the results are lactates of 4.0, 3.9 and 3.8 mmol/L.

What would be the most appropriate course of action?

Options

- A. Category 1 caesarean section.
- B. Category 2 caesarean section.
- C. Repeat sampling no more than 1 hour later if this is still indicated by the CTG trace, or sooner if additional nonreassuring or abnormal features are seen.
- D. Repeat sampling no more than 30 minutes later if this is still indicated by the CTG trace, or sooner if additional nonreassuring or abnormal features are seen.
- E. Trial of instrumental delivery in theatre.

90. A 35-year-old para 1 is referred from her community midwife to confirm presentation, as this is clinically uncertain. The fetus is cephalic, and she is offered a membrane sweep. The woman is unsure, as she has heard that this is painful, but is also keen to avoid postdates induction if possible. You advise her on the efficacy of membrane sweeping using the number needed to treat.

In how many women must a membrane sweep be performed to avoid one formal postdates induction?

Options

    A. 2.
    B. 3.
    C. 8.
    D. 15.
    E. 23.

91. You assist with the insertion of a cervical cerclage. The medical student observing asks about the indications for this procedure.

Which of the following women would be the best candidate for cervical cerclage?

Options

    A. A 25-year-old para 0 at 24^{+5} weeks' gestation, contracting with cervix 3 cm dilated.
    B. A 32-year-old para 1^{+1} (29-week preterm delivery, 12-week miscarriage) at 17 weeks' gestation with cervical funnelling and cervical length of 27 mm.
    C. A 32-year-old para 1^{+3} (28-week preterm labour) with twin pregnancy.
    D. A 34-year-old para 1^{+0} (30-week preterm delivery) with ultrasound cervical length of 25 mm at 18 weeks' gestation.
    E. A 40-year-old para 0 in vitro fertilization pregnancy with history of a previous cone biopsy.

92. A senior labour ward sister asks you to work with her updating your unit's guideline about whether mothers should be offered delivery on the midwife-led unit or the obstetric-led unit, both of which are on the same site. She is keen to ensure the unit is working to national guidance. All women arriving on the unit are first assessed in a triage area, unless delivery appears to be imminent, and then are directed to the obstetric labour ward or midwifery-led labour ward.

Which of the following women should be offered delivery on the midwife-led unit?

Options

A. A 29-year-old para 4 (SVDs) with a BMI of 24 in spontaneous labour. She has mild stable hypothyroidism on 100 mcg levothyroxine daily and there have been no antenatal problems. The cervix is 8 cm dilated on arrival, and the fetal heart is normal on auscultation.

B. A 34-year-old para 2 (SVDs) with a booking BMI of 36 presenting in spontaneous labour at 39^{+3} weeks' gestation. Serial fetal growth scans have revealed abdominal circumference between the 50th and 90th centile, with good growth. The cervix is 6 cm dilated and the CTG is normal.

C. A 34-year-old primigravida with a BMI of 34 is in spontaneous labour at 41^{+3} weeks' gestation. She has mild asthma and occasionally uses a salbutamol inhaler; the asthma seems to have improved over the last few years and she has had no hospital admissions. She is otherwise well and there have been no antenatal problems. She is 4 cm dilated and the fetal heart is normal on auscultation.

D. A healthy 21-year-old para 1 (previous caesarean section for breech presentation) has had a straightforward antenatal period and is keen for a vaginal birth after caesarean. She presents at 39^{+5} weeks' gestation in spontaneous labour. On examination the fetus is cephalic, the cervix is 9 cm dilated and the CTG is normal.

E. A healthy 25-year-old para 1 (SVD, followed by manual removal of placenta) who has had an unremarkable antenatal period presents in spontaneous labour at 40^{+3} weeks' gestation. The cervix is 7 cm dilated. The fetal heart is normal on auscultation.

93. A healthy 28-year-old low-risk, primigravid woman attends a routine antenatal appointment at 28 weeks with her midwife. The woman has always been keen to have a home delivery but wants to do what is safest for her baby. She also had a friend who was transferred to hospital in advanced labour, and the woman wants to avoid this. She asks her midwife if there is any increased risk to her baby from a home delivery compared with a planned delivery in an obstetric unit and what her chance of transfer to hospital in labour or immediately after delivery would be.

Which would be the best advice?

Options

- A. Approximately 10% increased relative risk of adverse perinatal outcome with a 35% chance of transfer.
- B. Approximately 30% increased relative risk of adverse perinatal outcome with 35% chance of transfer.
- C. Approximately 80% increased absolute risk of adverse perinatal outcome with 45% chance of transfer.
- D. Approximately 80% increased relative risk of adverse perinatal outcome with a 45% chance of transfer.
- E. No significant increased risk of perinatal mortality with a 10% chance of transfer.

94. A 40-year-old para 3 is delivered by SVD, and oxytocin 10 IU is given intramuscularly. During cord traction the woman screams in severe pain, the uterus is no longer palpable abdominally and the uterine fundus can be felt inverted in the vagina. The emergency buzzer is pressed.

What is the next immediate step that should be performed?

Options

- A. Administer tocolytic.
- B. Hydrostatic pressure with warm sodium chloride.
- C. Immediate manual replacement and simultaneous resuscitation.
- D. Immediate transfer to theatre for general anaesthetic and manual replacement in theatre.
- E. Verbal consent for Huntingdon's procedure.

ANSWERS

85. Answer: A.

Explanation: Misoprostol is an extremely strong uterotonic and is not licensed for use in pregnancy in the UK. It must be used with extreme caution in the second and third trimesters. Delivering these small doses accurately can be a challenge, as tablets need to be halved or quartered, but a pharmacist can help with suitable arrangements. Dissolving the tablet in water is often helpful.

References: MBRRACE-UK 2014: Lessons learned to inform future maternity care from the UK and Ireland Confidential Enquiries into Maternal Deaths and Morbidity 2009–2012.

Nzewi C, Araklitis G, Narvekar N (2014). The use of mifepristone and misoprostol in the management of late intrauterine fetal death. *The Obstetrician & Gynecologist* 16 (4), 233–238.

86. Answer: C.

Explanation: All women with IUFD should have TSH, FT$_3$ and FT$_4$ to check for occult maternal thyroid disease. The others are not part of routine initial investigations. Testing for alloimmune antiplatelet antibodies is indicated if fetal intracranial haemorrhage is found on postmortem. Anti-Ro and anti-La antibodies are appropriate if there is evidence of hydrops, endomyocardial fibroelastosis or atrioventricular node calcification at postmortem. Cocaine metabolites are only required if the history and presentation are suggestive of drug misuse. Parental karyotypes are indicated if fetal karyotype is suggestive of an unbalanced translocation, another fetal aneuploidy or if fetal genetic testing fails and the history is suggestive of aneuploidy.

Reference: Royal College of Obstetricians and Gynaecologists (2010). Green-top Guideline No. 55. Late intrauterine fetal death and stillbirth. London.

87. Answer: B.

Explanation: A number of meta-analyses have all concluded that STAN results in fewer episodes of fetal blood sampling and instrumental deliveries.

Reference: Sacco A, Muglu J, Navaratnarajah R, Hogg M (2015). ST analysis for intrapartum fetal monitoring. *The Obstetrician & Gynaecologist* 17 (1), 5–12.

88. Answer: A.

Explanation: Although airway adjuncts and supraglottic devices (such as laryngeal mask airway) may be suitable during cardiopulmonary resuscitation in the nonpregnant patient, especially for those inexperienced in intubation (many nonanaesthetist doctors in the UK), pregnant patients have an increased risk of regurgitation and aspiration, and definitive intubation should ideally be performed. In this case there is both an anaesthetist and an operating department practitioner present (commonly present in the UK and can assist the anaesthetist with intubation). A surgical airway is clearly not indicated here.

Reference: Royal College of Obstetricians and Gynaecologists (2011). Green-top Guideline No. 56. Maternal collapse in pregnancy and the puerperium. London.

89. Answer: C.

Explanation: This is a normal fetal blood sample result, and the labour is progressing well. Lactate or pH can be used in fetal blood sampling.

Lactate	pH	Interpretation
≤4.1	≥7.25	Normal
4.2–4.8	7.21–7.24	Borderline
≥4.9	≤7.20	Abnormal

Reference: National Institute of Clinical Excellence (2014). Clinical guideline 190. Intrapartum care: Care of healthy women and their babies during childbirth. London.

90. Answer: C.

Explanation: A Cochrane review in 2005 found the number needed to treat was 8.

Reference: Royal College of Obstetricians and Gynaecologists. StratOG, core training, management of labour and delivery.

91. Answer: D.

Explanation: This woman has a previous preterm labour and a cervical length on ultrasound of less than or equal to 25 mm. Given the risks of iatrogenic rupture of membranes, rescue cerclage is rarely indicated in affluent countries after 24 weeks' gestation. Cervical funnelling in the absence of a cervical length of less than or equal to 25 mm is not an indication for cerclage. Cerclage is not recommended in multiple pregnancies regardless of risk factors, although individualized decisions have to be made. Cone biopsy alone is not an indication for cerclage.

Reference: Royal College of Obstetricians and Gynaecologists (2011). Green-top Guideline 60. Cervical cerclage. London.

92. Answer: C.

Explanation: This woman has well-controlled, very mild asthma. Her age and BMI are less than 35 and she can therefore be considered 'low risk'. Women aged 35 years or older, with a BMI of over 35 or who are grand multiparous (para 4 or more), are at increased risk of postpartum haemorrhage and should deliver on an obstetric unit. A woman with previous manual removal of placenta is at increased risk of recurrence and should deliver on an obstetric unit. A woman with a previous caesarean section is at increased risk of uterine rupture and also of need for repeat caesarean section and should deliver on an obstetric unit with continuous electronic fetal monitoring.

Reference: National Institute of Clinical Excellence (2014). Clinical guideline 190. Intrapartum care: Care of healthy women and their babies during childbirth. London.

93. Answer: D.

Explanation: The Birthplace National Cohort Study was designed to answer questions about risks and benefits of giving birth in different settings in England, particularly for 'low-risk' women. The risk of adverse perinatal outcome is increased from 5.3 per 1000 to 9.3 per 1000 for a woman with a planned home delivery compared with a planned obstetric unit delivery for 'low-risk' nulliparous women. This is just under an 80% increased relative risk, but a 0.4% increased absolute risk. 'Low-risk' women should be offered a choice of planned place of birth, but it is important they are given relevant information to allow them to make an informed choice.

References: National Institute for Health and Care Excellence (2014). Clinical guideline 190. Intrapartum care: Care of healthy women and their babies during childbirth. London.

Birthplace in England Collaborative Group, et al. (2011). Perinatal and maternal outcomes by planned place of birth for healthy women with low risk pregnancies: The Birthplace in England National Prospective Cohort Study. *BMJ* 23, 343.

94. Answer: C.

Explanation: The first step is to attempt manual replacement; simultaneous resuscitation should be performed. If there are additional free staff, preparations for subsequent steps can also be made.

Reference. Bhalla R, et al. (2009). Acute inversion of the uterus. *The Obstetrician & Gynaecologist* 11 (1), 13–18.

Module 11   Management of the delivery

QUESTIONS

95. An F2 doctor is interested in obstetrics. He performs an SVD with the midwife, and he asks you to do a case-based discussion with him on the mechanisms of normal labour. You have a fetal skull model to help.

What is the length of the suboccipitobregmatic diameter?

Options

    A. 8.5 cm.
    B. 9.5 cm.
    C. 10 cm.
    D. 11.5 cm.
    E. 14 cm.

96. An obese 36-year-old primigravid Jehovah's Witness labours spontaneously at term. The fetal head is delivered but, with the next contraction, the midwife cannot deliver the shoulders. A shoulder dystocia is announced, and help is called for. The woman is put into McRoberts' position.

What is the next most appropriate immediate course of action?

Options

    A. Downward traction of fetus.
    B. Posterior axilla sling with a Foley catheter.
    C. Routine axial traction of fetus.
    D. Rubin II manoeuvre.
    E. Zanvanelli manoeuvre.

97. A senior obstetric trainee spends the day with an obstetric anaesthetist as part of his training in advanced labour ward practice. During a caesarean section the spinal block is not sufficiently effective, and a decision is made to perform a general anaesthetic.

What is the most commonly used induction agent in obstetric anaesthetic practice in the UK?

Options

- A. Isoflurane.
- B. Midazolam.
- C. Propofol.
- D. Suxamethonium.
- E. Thiopentone.

98. A pregnant woman walks into the A&E department and collapses; the collapse is witnessed by the receptionist. The patient is unresponsive and has no breathing or pulse. CPR is commenced immediately, and an emergency call goes out. The obstetric registrar arrives 3 minutes after CPR is commenced. Medical and anaesthetic teams are already performing the necessary advanced adult life support, including left uterine displacement. There is pulseless electrical activity, and adrenaline has been given. There are no notes or relatives with the woman, but there is a letter with an antenatal clinic appointment. This confirms she is 25 years old and pregnant. Her uterine fundus is above the maternal umbilicus. There is an ultrasound machine in the A&E. The team asks the obstetric registrar what additional measures should occur.

What important course of action should be taken in addition?

Options

- A. Initiate perimortem caesarean section in A&E after 4 minutes of CPR, aiming to deliver the fetus by 5 minutes since initiation of CPR.
- B. Initiate perimortem caesarean section in A&E after 5 minutes of CPR, aiming to deliver the fetus by 6 minutes since initiation of CPR.
- C. Phone obstetric consultant to discuss perimortem caesarean section.

D. Transfer to operating theatre for perimortem caesarean section as soon as possible.

E. Ultrasound to check for fetal heart, then perform perimortem caesarean section if the fetus is alive.

99. A 29-year-old para 2 with a booking BMI of 56 presents at 39^{+3} weeks' gestation in labour. She is found to be 4 cm dilated and contracting 3 : 10 regularly. The presentation is uncertain, and the obstetric ST3 is called to confirm fetal presentation. During the ultrasound the woman has a spontaneous rupture of membranes. Ultrasound suggests a footling breech presentation. On examination the woman is dysmorphic looking. Vaginal examination confirms 4 cm dilatation, but with a cord prolapse, and an emergency call is made. The ST3 anaesthetist and ST7 paediatrician attend immediately, and the midwife telephones the consultant obstetrician and anaesthetist to come in from home. The ST3 anaesthetist is concerned and alerts you to an antenatal assessment examination that includes 'Mallampati 3, thyromental distance 5 cm'. The CTG has a baseline rate of 140, variability greater than 5, no accelerations and variable decelerations with fast recovery lasting less than a minute with every contraction.

What would be the most appropriate immediate course of action?

Options

A. Continuous CTG, allow labour to progress and consider a fetal electrode.

B. Fill bladder with 750 ml saline, consider tocolysis, transfer to theatre and attempt regional anaesthetic for caesarean section.

C. Fill bladder with 750 ml saline, transfer to theatre and attempt regional anaesthetic for caesarean section.

D. Manually lift fetal head with immediate transfer to theatre for immediate general anaesthetic and category 1 caesarean section.

E. Manually replace cord, consider tocolysis and external cephalic version.

100. A 27-year-old primigravida from Somalia presents in labour, 5 cm dilated. The midwife suspects female genital mutilation (FGM) and, after discussion with the woman, confirms that this took place as a child. On examination there is evidence of clitoridectomy. The labia are fused together, having apparently been stitched together as a child leaving a small introitus. She explains that intercourse took numerous painful episodes before it was possible after her marriage. An epidural is given and a midline anterior episiotomy is performed. She goes on to have an SVD.

What type of FGM?

Options

    A. I.
    B. II.
    C. III.
    D. IV.
    E. Does not have FGM.

101. A 28-year-old primigravida spontaneously labours at 40^{+6} weeks' gestation. The first stage of labour is augmented at 5 cm labour and lasts for 11 hours. After 1 hour of passive second stage, she pushes for 2 hours and is exhausted. On examination the fetus is cephalic with 2/5 of the head palpable per abdomen. The cervix is fully dilated, direct OP position with 2+ caput, 3+ moulding and station −1. She is contracting strongly at 4:10. The CTG is normal, and the epidural is working well.

Which would be the best management?

Options

    A. Caesarean section.
    B. Continue pushing, reassess in 1 hour.
    C. Trial of OP delivery with nonrotational forceps in theatre.
    D. Trial of Keilland's forceps in theatre.
    E. Trial of rotational ventouse delivery in theatre.

102. A 33-year-old primigravida with an IVF pregnancy labours spontaneously at 38^{+6} weeks' gestation. Despite augmentation and good contractions her labour does not progress past 6 cm, and a category 2 caesarean section is arranged. The woman consents to caesarean but is distressed to be told that hysterectomy is a possible complication. She asks how common this is.

How would you best describe the frequency of caesarean hysterectomy?

Options

- A. Common.
- B. Rare.
- C. Uncommon.
- D. Very common.
- E. Very rare.

103. A 25-year-old para 1 is on her first day after a forceps delivery and is reviewed on the postnatal ward. She is obese, and the epidural in labour had been difficult. There were extensive vaginal tears that took some time to repair. She now complains of left foot drop with paraesthesia over the dorsum and calf over this side. Other than this, peripheral neurologic examination is normal, and she has been mobilizing.

What is the most likely cause?

Options

- A. Epidural haematoma.
- B. Neuropraxia to common peroneal nerve.
- C. Neuropraxia to pudendal nerve.
- D. Neurotmesis to common peroneal nerve.
- E. Neurotmesis to pudendal nerve.

104. A 32-year-old primigravida with paraplegia after a T5 spinal cord injury presents in spontaneous labour at 37^{+0} weeks' gestation having self-palpated her contractions. On examination the cervix is 6 cm dilated. Her BP is 102/68 mm Hg. Fifteen minutes later her BP is found to be 145/93 mm Hg. The CTG is normal.

What is the best immediate management?

Options

    A. Labetalol 200 mg orally.
    B. Nifedipine capsule 10 mg bite and swallow.
    C. Nifedipine modified release 10 mg orally.
    D. Nitroprusside.
    E. Observe BP.

Module 11   Management of the delivery

ANSWERS

95. Answer: B.

Explanation: This is the presenting diameter of a flexed OA delivery.

Reference: Royal College of Obstetricians and Gynaecologists. StratOG, core training, management of labour and delivery, mechanisms of normal labour and delivery.

96. Answer: C.

Explanation: Routine axial traction should be applied once the woman is in McRoberts' position. Downward traction increases the risk of brachial plexus injury and should be avoided. The other manoeuvres may be appropriate later.

Reference: Royal College of Obstetricians and Gynaecologists (2012). Green-top Guideline No. 42. Shoulder dystocia, 2nd ed. London.

97. Answer: E.

Explanation: Thiopentone and propofol are induction agents. Thiopentone is most commonly used due to extensive experience in caesarean deliveries. Midazolam would not normally be used as an inducing agent, and certainly not for caesarean section. Suxamethonium is a muscle relaxant. Isoflurane is a volatile gas. A very basic knowledge of obstetric anaesthesia is needed to help liaise effectively with anaesthetists.

Reference: Royal College of Obstetricians and Gynaecologists. Strat OG, core training, management of labour and delivery.

98. Answer: A.

Explanation: A perimortem caesarean section should now be initiated. As the fundus is above the umbilicus it can be presumed that gestation is greater than 20 weeks. Delivery of the fetus and placenta reduces oxygen consumption, improves venous return and cardiac output, facilitates chest compressions and makes ventilation easier. It should be performed regardless of viability or indeed whether the fetus is alive or dead. Although senior input should be sought at some point, it must not delay the urgently indicated management. Unnecessary transfer of the patient should also not delay delivery.

Reference: Royal College of Obstetricians and Gynaecologists (2011). Green-top Guideline No. 56. Maternal collapse in pregnancy and the puerperium. London.

99. Answer: B.

Explanation: This woman has a cord prolapse in the first stage of labour, and emergency caesarean section is indicated. She has a potentially very difficult airway as well as being operatively challenging. It would be prudent to ensure very experienced anaesthetic and obstetric presence before commencing caesarean section. The best course of action, therefore, would be to fill the bladder and consider a tocolytic. The anaesthetic team will probably be keen to attempt regional anaesthesia.

Reference: Royal College of Obstetricians and Gynaecologists (2014). Green-top Guideline No. 50. Umbilical cord prolapse. London.

100. Answer: C.

The World Health Organisation classification of female genital mutilation (FGM) describe Type 3 FGM as narrowing of the vaginal orifice with creation of a covering seal by cutting and appositioning the labia minora and/or the labia majora, with or without excision of the clitoris (infibulation).

Reference: Royal College of Obstetricians and Gynaecologists (2015). Green-top Guideline No. 53. Female genital mutilation and its management, 2nd ed. London.

101. Answer: A.

Explanation: This woman's labour is obstructed. It is not safe to perform operative vaginal delivery with 2/5 fetal head palpable and at station −1.

References: National Institute for Health and Care Excellence. (2014). Clinical guideline 190. Intrapartum care: Care of healthy women and their babies during childbirth. London.

Royal College of Obstetricians and Gynaecologists (2011). Green-top Guideline No. 26. Operative vaginal delivery, 3rd ed. London.

102. Answer: C.

Explanation: Uncommon. It is 7 to 8 per 1000, and 1 to 10 per 1000 can be described as uncommon.

Reference: Royal College of Obstetricians and Gynaecologists (2009). Consent Advice No. 7: caesarean section, 2nd ed. London.

103. Answer: B.

Explanation: Injury to the common peroneal nerve is most likely from prolonged hyperflexion of the thighs in lithotomy position. Neuropraxia is caused by external compression of the nerve and the prognosis is good, with recovery likely to be weeks or months. Although important to consider, epidural haematoma is very rare, and not in keeping with these examination findings. Neurotmesis, disruption of both the nerve and the nerve sheath, is unlikely.

Reference: Kuponiyi O, Alleemudder D, Latunde-Dada A, Eedarapalli P (2014). Nerve injuries associated with gynaecological surgery. *The Obstetrician & Gynaecologist* 16 (1), 29–36.

104. Answer: B.

Explanation: This woman is potentially developing autonomic dysreflexia, a potentially fatal medical emergency. The treatment involves removing the trigger, although this is not easily possible with labour. The most immediate thing to do is likely give nifedipine either bite and swallow or sublingually. The other antihypertensive agents are too slow acting.

Reference: Dawood R, Altanis E, Ribes-Pastor P, Ashworth F (2014). Pregnancy and spinal cord injury. *The Obstetrician & Gynaecologist* 16 (1), 99–107.

Module 12   Postnatal

QUESTIONS

105. A 27-year-old primigravida presents at 35^{+3} weeks' gestation with a headache and 24 hours of no fetal movement. An IUFD and preeclampsia are diagnosed. Induction of labour is performed. Four days after delivery her BP is still very labile, and she continues to require second-line oral therapy. She is troubled by lactation and breast pain.

What would be the best management for her?

Options

    A. Cabergoline.
    B. Bromocriptine.
    C. Metoclopramide.
    D. Ethinyl oestradiol.
    E. Simple measures such as supportive bra, ice packs and analgesia.

106. A 23-year-old medical student has delivered a healthy male neonate weighing 2900 g at term 36 hours ago by SVD. The mother is generally fit and well and has been granted a year out of her studies, having found out she was pregnant shortly after her elective in Papua New Guinea. She has noticed that, this morning, the neonate has rapidly developed severe bilateral conjunctivitis with a profuse purulent discharge. Last night the neonate's eyes looked normal.

What is the most likely causative organism in this case of neonatal conjunctivitis?

Options

    A. *Chlamydia trachomatis.*
    B. Herpes simplex virus type 1.
    C. HPV type 6.
    D. *Neisseria gonorrhoeae.*
    E. *Trichomonas vaginalis.*

107. A 32-year-old primigravida commences a planned delivery in a rural stand-alone midwifery unit. After 8 hours of established labour, the second stage of labour is diagnosed. The woman develops an urge to push 1 hour later and she commences pushing. After 30 minutes late decelerations are heard on intermittent auscultation. On examination the fetus is cephalic, 2/5 palpable per abdomen, fully dilated, direct OP and at station spines −1. There is 3+ caput and 3+ moulding. A decision is made for transfer to hospital, although this is delayed because of treacherous snow-covered and ice-covered roads. On arrival at hospital 3 hours later the CTG is severely abnormal, with examination findings unchanged and a category 1 caesarean section is performed. Ten minutes after delivery resuscitation is stopped for a few seconds while the neonate is reassessed. The fetus is still extremely floppy, with no pulse, no response to stimulation and no spontaneous breathing. It is blue.

What is the infant's 10-minute Apgar score?

Options

    A. 0.
    B. 1.
    C. 2.
    D. 3.
    E. 4.

108. A 32-year-old obese primigravida has a forceps delivery at 39^{+2} weeks' gestation for suspected fetal compromise. Because the baby is not spontaneously crying at delivery, the obstetrician clamps and cuts the cord immediately. Shortly afterwards, however, the baby spontaneously cries after stimulation by the midwife. The following day the baby feeds poorly and is found to be anaemic. The issue of cord clamping in term neonates is discussed and debated between the obstetricians and neonatologists at the next perinatal morbidity meeting.

What is the best management regarding cord clamping in term neonates?

Options

    A. Cord clamping 1 to 5 minutes postdelivery unless infant heart rate is less than 60 bpm or there is concern about the integrity of the cord, followed by oxytocin 10 IU intramuscularly (IM).

    B. Cord clamping 1 to 5 minutes postdelivery unless infant heart rate is less than 100 bpm or there is concern about the integrity of the cord, followed by oxytocin 10 IU IM.

    C. Cord clamping 1 to 5 minutes postdelivery unless infant is not spontaneously crying or there is concern about the integrity of the cord, followed by oxytocin 10 IU IM.

    D. Oxytocin 10 IU IM at delivery of neonate, cord clamping 1 to 5 minutes postdelivery unless infant heart rate is less than 60 bpm or there is concern about the integrity of the cord.

    E. Oxytocin 10 IU IM at delivery of neonate, cord clamping 1 to 5 minutes postdelivery unless infant heart rate is less than 100 bpm or there is concern about the integrity of the cord.

109. A healthy 34-year-old low-risk primigravida is referred to the obstetric antenatal clinic by her midwife at the woman's request to discuss the management of the third stage of labour. Her antenatal group has advised her to have physiological management of the third stage of labour to improve bonding with her baby. They suggest that, as long as she delivers in a quiet room, her own endogenous oxytocin will work well and, as she is 'low risk'; her chance of postpartum haemorrhage will be no higher than if she were to have an active management of the third stage. The woman asks you for your advice and rationale for this regarding management of her third stage of labour.

Which is the best advice?

Options

    A. Advise her there is no difference in outcome between active management and physiological management of third stage of labour. Because she is low risk, either are appropriate choices.

    B. Recommend active management of third stage of labour, because it is associated with a slightly decreased risk of haemorrhage and blood transfusion compared with physiological third stage.

    C. Recommend active management of third stage of labour, because it is associated with approximately half the risk of haemorrhage of more than 1 L and approximately a third of blood transfusion compared with physiological third stage.

    D. Recommend controlled cord traction, because it is associated with shorter third stage and higher maternal satisfaction, but there is no need for oxytocin as she is low risk.

    E. Recommend physiological management of third stage, converting to active management if there is a delay in the delivery of the placenta.

110. A 32-year-old low-risk primigravida presents with contractions at 26^{+0} weeks' gestation. On examination the cervix is 5 cm dilated. She is admitted, steroids are given and a magnesium sulphate infusion is commenced. She is anxious and is keen to know a very approximate prognosis for her fetus.

Approximately what percentage of live births at 26 weeks' gestation will go on to survive without disability?

Options

    A. 10%.
    B. 15%.
    C. 20%.
    D. 60%.
    E. 90%.

111. A 33-year-old primigravida with asthma delivers a live infant at term. There was no meconium. The infant makes no spontaneous attempt at breathing and is floppy. It is dried, covered and assessed. Five inflation breaths are performed. There is good chest movement on inflation. The neonate is then reassessed: there is a heart rate of around 50 bpm although still no breathing. Senior assistance is summoned and en route.

What is the next immediate step?

Options

    A. Chest compressions and ventilation breaths in ratio 1:1.
    B. Chest compressions and ventilation breaths in ratio 3:1.
    C. Chest compressions and ventilation breaths in ratio 5:1.
    D. Chest compressions and ventilation breaths in ratio 15:1.
    E. Chest compressions and ventilation breaths in ratio 30:2.

112. A 34-year-old primigravida has a water birth. There is significant perineal trauma. On examination the external anal sphincter is completely severed, as is the internal anal sphincter, although the rectal mucosa is intact.

What classification of perineal tear is this?

Options

    A. 3a.
    B. 3b.
    C. 3c.
    D. 3d.
    E. 4.

113. A 35-year-old now para 1 attends for perineal review after an episiotomy wound infection 1 week postdelivery. All has healed well. She has had difficulties with a variety of contraceptive methods she has tried over a number of years and is keen to rely on lactational amenorrhoea. She asks about its efficacy.

If a mother is amenorrhoeic, is less than 6 months postnatal and is exclusively breast feeding, how effective is lactational amenorrhoea as a method of contraception?

Options

    A. 90%.
    B. 92%.
    C. 94%.
    D. 96%.
    E. 98%.

114. A 25-year-old para 5 is due to get a LNG-IUS inserted 4 weeks post caesarean section. She defaults the appointment due to child care, but attends 3 weeks later (7 weeks postnatally). She is formula feeding her infant. She remains amenorrhoeic and had sexual intercourse with her husband 2 weeks previously, but has not since because it was too uncomfortable. A pregnancy test is negative. She is very keen for contraception, ideally with LNG-IUS, but does not want a progesterone implant.

What would be the best management?

Options

    A. Advise condoms or abstinence, bring back in 1 week and insert LNG-IUS if pregnancy test negative.

    B. Advise condoms or abstinence, bring back in 2 weeks and insert LNG-IUS if pregnancy test negative.

    C. Give depot medroxyprogesterone acetate, bring back in 2 weeks and insert LNG-IUS.

    D. Insert copper (Cu)-IUS.

    E. Insert LNG-IUS.

115. A 37-year-old para 1 had significant gestational hypertension in her last few weeks of antenatal care. Postnatally the BP has not been under control despite maximum dose labetalol. She suffered intolerable side effects from nifedipine and is therefore commenced on an ACE inhibitor. She is breast feeding and is keen for something safe for her infant.

Which of these ACE inhibitors has the most infant safety data in breast feeding?

Options

    A. Enalapril.

    B. Imidapril.

    C. Lisinopril.

    D. Perindopril.

    E. Ramipril.

116. You are called to an emergency cardiac arrest on the labour ward. An F2 doctor was inserting a new cannula into a 29-year-old 70 kg woman 2 hours postnatally and has flushed the cannula with 10 ml of 1% lidocaine instead of 0.9% NaCl. Cardiopulmonary resuscitation (CPR) has been commenced by the time of your arrival.

What should be injected immediately into this woman while CPR is taking place?

Options

    A. 0.5 ml 1:10,000 adrenaline (50 mcg) IV.
    B. 10 ml 10% calcium carbonate slow IV.
    C. 10 ml 10% calcium gluconate slow IV.
    D. 100 ml intralipid 10% IV over 1 minute.
    E. 100 ml intralipid 20% IV over 1 minute.

117. A 36-year-old primigravida has an emergency caesarean section for failure to progress following a long period of augmentation and delivers a 4.8 kg baby. Despite various uterotonics, the uterus remains hypotonic and there is bleeding. The haemorrhage stops temporarily with compression. A decision to perform a B-Lynch suture is performed. A suture on a large needle is requested.

Which would be the best suture material to use?

Options

    A. Poliglecaprone 25 1.
    B. Poliglecaprone 25 2-0.
    C. Polydiaxone 1.
    D. Polyglactin 910 1-0.
    E. Polyglactin 910 2-0.

118. A 28-year-old para 1 who is keen to breast feed is being debriefed after her caesarean section the previous day. She has had a variety of complex mental health issues and you discuss her management with the psychiatrist who has come to visit her on the ward.

Which of the following drugs is the safest for the infant if the mother is breast feeding?

Options

    A. Carbamazapine.
    B. Citalopram.
    C. Clozapine.
    D. Lithium.
    E. Phenobarbital.

119. You are attending a regional annual perinatal morbidity and mortality meeting.

How is perinatal mortality in the UK defined?

Options

    A. The number of fetal and neonatal deaths from 24 weeks' gestation to 7 days postnatal per 1000 live births.
    B. The number of fetal and neonatal deaths from 24 weeks' gestation to 7 days postnatal per 10,000 live births.
    C. The number of fetal and neonatal deaths from 24 weeks' gestation to 28 days postnatal per 1000 live births.
    D. The number of fetal and neonatal deaths from 24 weeks' gestation to 28 days postnatal per 10,000 live births.
    E. The number of fetal and neonatal deaths from 24 weeks' gestation to 7 days postnatal per 100,000 live births.

Module 12   Postnatal

ANSWERS

105. Answer: E.

Explanation: Dopamine agonists can be successful in suppressing lactation (cabergoline is superior to bromocriptine); both, however, are contraindicated in women with hypertension. Oestrogen increases the thromboembolic risk, is of unproven benefit for lactation suppression and should not be used. Metoclopramide is also a dopamine antagonist and has been used to promote lactation, although evidence of effectiveness is poor and it is not commonly used for this indication in the UK. Nonpharmacologic measures alone therefore are the only reasonable option in this woman.

Reference: Royal College of Obstetricians and Gynaecologists (2010). Green-top Guideline No. 55. Late intrauterine fetal death and stillbirth. London.

106. Answer: D.

Explanation: This neonate probably has neonatal conjunctivitis secondary to gonorrhoea, which he has contracted from the mother's genital tract during delivery. Gonorrhoea infection typically results in a rapidly developing severe conjunctivitis associated with a profuse purulent discharge within 48 hours of birth. Neonatal conjunctivitis secondary to chlamydia typically presents day 5 to 14 postnatally with a less purulent discharge.

Reference: National Institute of Clinical Excellence. Clinical knowledge summaries, neonatal conjunctivitis. http://cks.nice.org.uk/conjunctivitis-infective#!scenario:2. Accessed January 2016.

107. Answer: A.

Explanation:

	0	**1**	**2**
Activity	Absent	Arms and legs flexed	Active movements
Pulse	Absent	<100	>100
Grimace	No response to stimulation	Grimace	Sneeze, cough, cry
Appearance	Blue or pale	Body pink, blue extremities	Pink all over
Respiration	Absent	Slow, irregular	Regular

References: Royal College of Obstetricians and Gynaecologists. StratOG, core training, postpartum and neonatal problems.

Apgar, V (1953). A proposal for a new method of evaluation of the newborn infant. *Current Researches in Anesthesia and Analgesia* 32 (4), 260–267.

108. Answer: D.

Explanation: Women should be recommended active management of third stage, with cord clamping advice as in D followed by controlled cord traction. The placenta should be delivered within 30 minutes of delivery.

Reference: National Institute of Clinical Excellence (2014). Clinical guideline 190. Intrapartum care: Care of healthy women and their babies during childbirth. London.

109. Answer: C.

Explanation: Active management of third stage should be advised to all women for the previously discussed reasons. Controlled cord traction should not be performed before oxytocin administration because of the risk of uterine inversion.

Reference: National Institute for Health and Care Excellence (2014). Clinical guideline 190. Intrapartum care: Care of healthy women and their babies during childbirth. London.

110. Answer: D.

Explanation: Although detailed discussions of prognosis should be individualized with neonatologists, it is important to know approximate prognosis of preterm deliveries. The EPICure studies have provided this information in the UK.

Reference: Moore T, et al. (2012). Neurological and developmental outcome in extremely preterm children born in England in 1995 and 2006: The EPICure studies. *BMJ* 345, e7961.

111. Answer: B.

Explanation: Chest compressions and ventilation breaths in ratio 3 : 1.

Reference: Richmond S, Wylie J (2010). Resuscitation Council (UK) resuscitation guideline 11. Neonatal life support. Available at: www.resus.org.uk. Accessed January 2016.

112. Answer: C.

Explanation: A 3d tear does not exist.

Reference: Royal College of Obstetricians and Gynaecologists (2015). Green-top Guideline No. 29. Third and Fourth degree tears, management, 3rd ed. London.

113. Answer: E.

Explanation: This relies on strictly meeting the criteria.

Reference: Faculty of Sexual and Reproductive Healthcare Clinical Guidance (2009). Postnatal sexual and reproductive health. London.

114. Answer: A.

Explanation: As this woman is now greater than 4 weeks postnatal and not breast feeding, and she has had sexual intercourse 2 weeks ago, one cannot be certain that she is not pregnant. Insertion of an IUD or IUS is therefore contraindicated, as is injecting depot medroxyprogesterone acetate. Although A or B are both safe, she is a relatively young grandmultipara and it would seem prudent to insert the LNG-IUS at the first safe opportunity.

Reference: Faculty of Sexual and Reproductive Healthcare Clinical Guidance (2009). Postnatal sexual and reproductive health. London.

115. Answer: A.

Explanation: Enalapril and captopril have no known adverse effects on infants receiving breast milk, and there is insufficient evidence about other ACE inhibitors. She should be advised to change to an alternative preparation if she is planning a further pregnancy.

References: National Institute of Clinical Excellence (2010). Clinical guideline 107. The management of hypertensive disorders in pregnancy. London.

Smith M, Waugh J, Nelson-Piercy C (2013). Management of postpartum hypertension. *The Obstetrician & Gynaecologist* 15 (1) 45–50.

116. Answer: E.

Explanation: Intralipid 20% IV 1.5 ml/kg over 1 minute is needed immediately in cases of collapse secondary to local anaesthetic toxicity; this should be followed by an infusion of 0.25 ml/kg/min. Calcium gluconate is used in magnesium sulphate toxicity, or in hyperkalaemia. Adrenaline 1 mg IV (1 ml 1:1000) is used during cardiopulmonary resuscitation as part of advanced life support. Although the optimum dose of adrenaline to use in cardiac arrest is unknown, 50 mcg IV is significantly lower than the recommended dose.

References: Royal College of Obstetricians and Gynaecologists (2011). Green-top Guideline No. 56. Maternal collapse in pregnancy and the puerperium. London.

The Association of Anaesthetists of Great Britain and Ireland Safety Guideline (2010). Management of severe local anaesthetic toxicity.

Resuscitation Council (UK) Advanced Life Support 2010.

117. Answer: A.

Explanation: The B-Lynch is a haemostatic suture used for postpartum haemorrhage to stop the bleeding without performing hysterectomy. The procedure was first described using number 2 chromic catgut but, with newer suture materials available, number 1 poliglecaprone 25 (Monocryl), an absorbable monofilament, is recommended. A 2-0 suture would be too thin for the strength required. It is important to know the generic names in addition to brand names of the common suture materials.

Reference: Allam MS (2005). B-Lynch C. *International Journal of Gynecology and Obstetrics* 89, 236–241.

118. Answer: B.

Explanation: Citalopram is excreted in the breast milk and may be used with caution if the benefits of breast feeding are likely to outweigh the risks. A woman who is on any of the other drugs should usually be advised not to breast feed.

Reference: National Institute of Clinical Excellence (2014). Clinical guideline 192. Antenatal and postnatal mental health: Clinical management and service guidance. London.

119. Answer: A.

Explanation: The number of fetal and neonatal deaths from 24 weeks' gestation to 7 days postnatal per 1000 live births.

Reference: MBRRACE-UK collaboration. Perinatal Mortality Surveillance Report: UK Perinatal Deaths for Births from January to December 2013. University of Leicester. 2015.

Module 13   Gynaecology

QUESTIONS

120. A 58-year-old postmenopausal woman presents for HRT counselling. While questioning her about her health, you ask her about the risk factors for osteoporosis from the fracture risk assessment (FRAX) tool, which is used to determine which individuals warrant further evaluation for osteoporosis by bone mineral density testing.

Which of the following is not part of the FRAX tool?

Options

- A.   Past smoking history.
- B.   Prior fracture as an adult.
- C.   Alcohol intake.
- D.   History of type 1 diabetes mellitus.
- E.   Paternal or maternal history of hip fractures.

121. A 56-year-old woman with a BMI of 38 and type 2 diabetes mellitus presents with daily dark brown staining on her underwear for the past week. She underwent menopause at age 53 and has had no further bleeding or discharge since that time. There has been no vaginal or vulval trauma, and her cervical smear test 6 months previously was normal. On examination her cervix appears normal and there is no evidence of external haemorrhoids. A urine dipstick test is negative for blood.

What is the next best step in the management of this patient?

Options

- A.   Dilatation and curettage.
- B.   Outpatient hysteroscopy.
- C.   Pipelle biopsy.
- D.   Transvaginal ultrasound.
- E.   Vabra biopsy.

122. A 39-year-old para 2 presents with a 3-year history of heavy painful periods in a 7/28 cycle. The onset of the heavy bleeding started after her laparoscopic tubal occlusion. She has a BMI of 39 and currently smokes 10 per day. She is also known to have type 2 diabetes and is hypertensive on beta blockers.

What is the most appropriate management option?

Options

    A. Abdominal hysterectomy.
    B. Endometrial ablation.
    C. Levonorgestrel-containing intrauterine device.
    D. Progesterone-only pills.
    E. Tranexamic acid.

123. A 35-year-old para 3 underwent a TAH+BSO for severe pelvic endometriosis that had not responded to medical and conservative surgical treatment. She attends for her follow-up appointment complaining of hot flushes and sweating.

Which HRT regime should you consider?

Options

    A. Combined continuous oestrogen/progestogen.
    B. Oestradiol patches.
    C. Oral oestradiol valerate.
    D. Progesterone-only HRT.
    E. Topical oestriol.

124. A 17-year-old girl presents with crampy lower abdominal pain which radiates to her legs. For the past year the pain has coincided with the first 3 days of her menses. She is not sexually active. Her history and general examination are unremarkable.

What is the optimum management approach?

Options

    A. Nonsteroidal antiinflammatory drugs.
    B. Combined oral contraceptives.
    C. Laparoscopic uterine nerve ablation.
    D. Progesterone-only pills in a continuous fashion.
    E. Transcutaneous nerve stimulation.

125. A 25-year-old patient presents with sudden-onset LIF pain associated with nausea and vomiting. She is sexually active, uses the Mirena intrauterine contraceptive device for contraception and is otherwise healthy. On examination she is tachycardic, and abdominal examination demonstrates tenderness over LIF with no rebound. Pelvic examination shows a normal cervix with no abnormal discharge, but fullness and tenderness on the left adnexa on bimanual examination. The urine pregnancy test is negative.

What is the most likely diagnosis?

Options

    A. Diverticulitis.
    B. Ectopic pregnancy.
    C. Ovarian torsion.
    D. Ruptured corpus luteum.
    E. Tubo-ovarian abscess.

126. A 28-year-old para 3 presents with vulval pruritus and burning. She reports dyspareunia and copious foul-smelling green vaginal discharge. On examination there is erythema of the vulva as well as petechiae of the upper vagina and cervix.

What is the most likely diagnosis?

Options

    A. Chlamydia.
    B. Gonorrhoea.
    C. Syphilis.
    D. *Trichomonas vaginalis.*
    E. Candidiasis.

127. A 25-year-old para 0, who has recently become sexually active, is complaining of new onset vulval pain. She describes pain with light touch, particularly on intercourse and when using tampons, and she localizes it to around the vulva. The pain is not present at other times. She does not report any itching, soreness or unusual discharge.

What is the most likely diagnosis?

Options

    A. Lichen sclerosus et atrophicus.
    B. Candidiasis.
    C. Vestibulodynia.
    D. Vulval endometriosis.
    E. Vulvodynia.

128. You are seeing a 62-year-old patient for a follow-up visit. You evaluated her for fracture risk 2 weeks ago and, given that she has high risk for fracture, you sent her for a DEXA scan. Her T score for bone mineral density in the hip was less than −2.5 and the thoracic spine less than −2.0. She has no secondary causes of osteoporosis, has not been on glucocorticoids recently, is a nonsmoker, and does not drink alcohol. There is no dysphagia, and she is able to sit upright for 1 hour after taking medications. It is determined that she should be placed on a bisphosphonate for treatment of her osteoporosis of the hip.

Which of the following does not affect the risk of fracture of the hip?

Options

    A. Alendronate.
    B. Etidronate.
    C. Risendronate.
    D. Zoledronic acid.
    E. None of the above.

129. A 24-year-old para 1 presents with a 6-hour history of right lower quadrant (RLQ) pain described as intermittent, severe in nature and associated with nausea and vomiting. She denies a change in bowel habits, and she is currently menstruating. On examination she is mildly tachycardic and has tenderness in the RLQ. Her urine pregnancy test is negative, and urine dipstick is negative for both blood and white cells. On pelvic examination she has a normal looking cervix, normal-sized and nontender uterus and no cervical motion tenderness. There is a palpable mass in the right adnexa which is tender to palpation and somewhat reproduces her pain. A transvaginal ultrasound shows a normal uterus and left ovary, but the right ovary measures 7 × 5 cm with cystic and solid components as well as with calcification. Colour flow Doppler is inconclusive.

What is the next best step in the management of this patient?

Options

    A. Laparoscopy.
    B. Laparotomy.
    C. Magnetic resonance imaging.
    D. Observation and symptom relief.
    E. Repeat transvaginal ultrasound scan.

130. Which of the following has been shown to contribute to surgical patients' enhanced recovery?

Options

    A. Allowing free fluids up to 1 hour before anaesthetic.
    B. Allowing free fluids up to 2 hours before anaesthetic.
    C. Allowing free fluids up to 6 hours before anaesthetic.
    D. Allowing free fluids up to 12 hours before anaesthetic.
    E. Mechanical bowel preparation.

131. Considering prophylactic oophorectomy at the time of hysterectomy for benign disease:

At what age is there no significant difference in survival in women at low/average risk for ovarian cancer?

Options

    A. 50 years.
    B. 55 years.
    C. 60 years.
    D. 65 years.
    E. 70 years.

132. A 25-year-old patient suffers with headaches, mood swings, irritability, depression and feeling out of control just before, and during, her menses. She also reports physical symptoms including breast tenderness, bloating and headaches. Her physical and psychological symptoms resolve completely after menstruation ceases.

Which of the following would be the best first-line management?

Options

    A. A second-generation combined oral contraceptive pill used cyclically.
    B. CBT.
    C. Continuous high-dose SSRI.
    D. Danazol.
    E. Vitamin B_6 20 mg daily.

133. A 29-year-old patient is undergoing a laparoscopic ovarian cystectomy for endometriosis. She is 170 cm tall and weighs 70 kg.

Which antibiotic regime should be adopted to reduce surgical site infection?

Options

    A. No antibiotics needed for prophylaxis.

    B. IV cefalexin 1.5 g at induction of anaesthesia.

    C. IV cefalexin 1.5 g and metronidazole 500 mg at induction of anaesthesia.

    D. IV metronidazole 500 mg at induction of anaesthesia.

    E. Intramuscular gentamicin 360 mg over 30 minutes.

134. A 24-year-old patient presents with vulval itching, soreness, vaginal discharge, and occasional dysuria. She has had thrush treatment at least five times over the previous 12 months for similar symptoms, with genital swabs confirming the diagnosis. A vaginal swab of vaginal discharge collected from the anterior fornix showed spores/pseudohyphae.

The recommended management approach is?

Options

    A. Clotrimazole pessary 500 mg weekly × 1 month.

    B. Clotrimazole pessary 500 mg weekly × 6 months.

    C. Fluconazole 100 mg weekly × 1 month.

    D. Fluconazole 100 mg weekly × 3 month.

    E. Metronidazole 400 mg orally twice a day for 5 to 7 days.

135. A 16-year-old girl presents with primary amenorrhoea. She has reached Tanner V breast and pubic hair development and, on pelvic examination, there is a blind ending vagina. The karyotype shows 46XX.

What is the most likely diagnosis?

Options

    A. Congenital adrenal hyperplasia.

    B. Constitutional delay.

    C. Mayer–Rokitansky–Küster-Hauser syndrome.

    D. McCune–Albright syndrome.

    E. Complete androgen insensitivity syndrome.

136. A 12-year-old girl presents to the A&E department with lower abdominal pain. On examination there is a large pelvi-abdominal mass. Transabdominal ultrasound scan shows bilateral solid ovarian tumours.

What is the most likely diagnosis?

Options

- A. Benign epithelial tumour.
- B. Epithelial ovarian cancer.
- C. Mature cystic teratoma.
- D. Ovarian fibroadenoma.
- E. Sex cord tumour.

137. In operative hysteroscopy, fluid distension is preferred over gas so that:

Options

- A. Bipolar energy can be used.
- B. There is less miscibility with blood and tissue debris.
- C. There is higher risk of intravasation of the medium.
- D. There is less risk of systemic absorption.
- E. It distends the field of view at low pressure.

138. In operative hysteroscopy, which of the following distension media has a risk of hyperglycaemia in fluid overload?

Options

- A. 1.5% glycine.
- B. 3% sorbitol.
- C. 5% mannitol.
- D. Dextran 70.
- E. Normal saline 0.9%.

139. A 70-year-old Caucasian patient was referred with a 2-year history of vulval and vaginal soreness unrelieved by vaginal oestrogen. She also reports recent onset dyspareunia, both superficial and deep. On further questioning she describes constipation, dysuria and both oral inflammation and ulceration. The examination confirmed oral ulceration and a white lacy pattern on the vulva. The vagina was very erythematous with a narrowed introitus and thin filmy adhesions to the mid-third.

The examination was extremely painful.

What is the most likely diagnosis?

Options

    A. Lichen planus.
    B. Lichen sclerosus et atrophicus.
    C. Lichen simplex.
    D. Menopausal atrophy.
    E. Psoriasis.

140. A 25-year-old para 2 presents with a 4-year history of progressive facial hirsutism and increasingly irregular periods. She had menarche at the age of 8. On examination she has moderately severe hirsutism on the face and chin and was not Cushingoid in appearance. Her BP was 136/83 mm Hg and her BMI was 23.3 kg/m^2. She reports that she was a tall child and volunteered that she has always had a small vaginal introitus with clitoromegaly and, since puberty, a high libido.

What are you likely to find in her laboratory blood tests?

Options

    A. Decreased serum testosterone.
    B. Elevated sex hormone-binding globulin.
    C. Elevated gonadotropins.
    D. Elevated 17-hydroxyprogesterone.
    E. Elevated TSH.

141. A 50-year-old patient is due to have a major abdominal surgery. She is currently taking combined continuous HRT for vasomotor symptoms.

When should she stop HRT before surgery?

Options

- A. 2 weeks.
- B. 4 weeks.
- C. 6 weeks.
- D. 8 weeks.
- E. 10 weeks.

142. A 55-year-old patient presents with severely debilitating vasomotor symptoms. She was declined HRT treatment by her general practitioner as her mother had had a PE while taking the combined oral contraceptive pills. She is otherwise fit and well with no significant previous medical or surgical history and has never had any gynaecologic surgery.

Which HRT would give her the lowest risk of VTE?

Options

- A. Screen for thrombophilia.
- B. LNG-IUS
- C. Oral combined continuous HRT.
- D. Oral combined sequential HRT.
- E. Transdermal combined HRT preparation.

143. In 2013 the International Ovarian Tumour Analysis Group (IOTA) published the largest study investigating the use of ultrasound to differentiate between benign and malignant ovarian masses. The group developed simple ultrasound rules.

Which of the following rules would NOT suggest a malignant process?

Options

- A. Ascites.
- B. At least four papillary structures.
- C. Irregular solid tumour.
- D. Presence of acoustic shadowing.
- E. Very strong blood flow.

144. A 15-year-old girl attended with her mother asking for the HPV vaccine as she missed the school immunization programme.

What does she need to do next?

Options

- A. There is no need to give the vaccine as she is beyond the vaccination age.
- B. She needs 2 doses of the vaccine 1 month apart.
- C. She needs 2 doses of the vaccine 6 months apart.
- D. She needs 3 doses of the vaccine with the second dose 1 month after and the third dose 6 months from first dose.
- E. She needs 3 doses of the vaccine 6 months apart.

145. A 35-year-old para 2 presents with dysmenorrhoea over the preceding 12 months. She also reports some dyschesia (difficultly defecating) during her periods. A transvaginal ultrasound scan confirmed a 7-cm endometrioma. She undergoes a laparoscopic ovarian cystectomy and excision of pelvic endometriosis.

Which is of the following should be your postsurgical management plan?

Options

- A. COCPs for 3 months.
- B. COCPs for 3 to 6 months.
- C. LNG-IUS for 18 months.
- D. GnRH for 6 months.
- E. GnRH for 12 months with add back tibolone.

146. A 60-year-old para 4 on a continuous combined HRT regimen presents with a 2-week history of irregular vaginal bleeding.

What is the most appropriate next step in her management?

Options

- A. Dilatation and curettage.
- B. Norethisterone 5 mg tid.
- C. Pipelle endometrial biopsy.
- D. Sequential combined HRT.
- E. Transvaginal ultrasound.

147. A 35-year-old patient presents 6 months after a normal vaginal delivery. The pregnancy was uncomplicated but, following delivery, a piece of placenta was apparently retained in the uterus. She was treated with antibiotics and later underwent a dilatation and curettage procedure. Now she presents with amenorrhoea. She is no longer breast feeding and is concerned.

What is the most appropriate next step in her management?

Options

    A. Hysterosalpingo-contrast sonography.
    B. Hysterosalpingogram.
    C. Hysteroscopy.
    D. Hysterosonography.
    E. Saline sonography.

148. A 45-year-old patient presents to the A&E department 2 days after UAE for a 20-weeks' size fibroid uterus. She has diffuse abdominal pain, generalized malaise, anorexia, nausea, vomiting, low-grade fever and leucocytosis.

What is the most likely diagnosis?

Options

    A. Arterial dissection.
    B. Bowel perforation.
    C. Endometritis.
    D. Myoma expulsion.
    E. Postembolization syndrome.

149. The fluid (1.5% glycine) deficit during an operative hysteroscopy using monopolar diathermy is calculated at 1000 ml.

What is the most appropriate step of action?

Options

    A. Abandon the procedure.
    B. Ask anaesthetist to site a central line.
    C. Complete the procedure as expeditiously as possible.
    D. Serum electrolyte values should be obtained and abnormalities managed appropriately.
    E. Start prophylactic seizure control drugs.

Module 13   Gynaecology

ANSWERS

120. Answer: A.

Explanation: The World Health Organization recommends the use of the FRAX tool to determine which women are at high risk of fracture over the forthcoming 10 years. Both the UK and the United States use this tool to help determine who needs further evaluation of bone mineral density of the hip and the lumbar spine. 'Current smoking' is among the questions in the FRAX tool, although 'past history of smoking' is not. Clinical judgment should be used, however, for those women with large numbers of pack-years of smoking and who only recently discontinued smoking. Prior fracture as an adult, which only includes those fractures that would not have occurred in an otherwise healthy adult woman, is included. Of women with osteopenia, Colles' fracture of the wrist in younger women and hip fracture in older women are most common. Alcohol intake plays a role in the nutritional status and fall risk in older women. Secondary risks for osteoporosis include type 1 diabetes, hyperthyroidism, premature ovarian failure, malabsorption, chronic liver disease, among others, and a parental history of hip fracture. Follow-up with DEXA scanning is warranted in those women deemed at high risk.

References: Kwun S, Laufgraben MJ, Gopalakrishnan G (2012). Prevention and treatment of postmenopausal osteoporosis. *The Obstetrician & Gynecologist* 14, 251–256.

WHO Fracture Risk Assessment Tool. Available from: http://www.shef.ac.uk/FRAX/tool.jsp.

121. Answer: D.

Explanation: Approximately 10% of women who are menopausal will develop postmenopausal bleeding within the first few years of their last menses. The first step in evaluation is transvaginal ultrasound to assess the endometrial thickness. An endometrial thickness less than 5 mm has 96% sensitivity for detecting endometrial cancer with a 39% false-positive rate. Unless bleeding recurs, a patient with an endometrial thickness less than 5 mm needs no further evaluation at this point. Hysteroscopy and biopsy play a role in recurrent symptoms or in those women with an endometrial thickness of 5 mm or greater. Dilatation and curettage in isolation is no longer indicated in the management of postmenopausal bleeding.

Reference: Bakour SH, Timmerman A, Mol BW, et al. (2012). Management of women with postmenopausal bleeding: Evidence-based review. *The Obstetrician & Gynaecologist* 14, 243–249.

122. Answer: C.

Explanation: Although endometrial ablation would be very reasonable, an anaesthetic is likely to be required, and this is not without risks given her comorbidities.

123. Answer: A.

Explanation: In women with surgically induced menopause because of endometriosis, combined oestrogen/progestogen therapy or tibolone can be effective in the treatment of menopausal symptoms. The European Society of Human Reproduction and Embryology guidelines recommend that, in postmenopausal women after hysterectomy and with a history of endometriosis, clinicians should avoid unopposed oestrogen treatment. The theoretical benefit of avoiding disease reactivation and malignant transformation of residual disease, however, should be balanced against the increased systemic risks associated with combined oestrogen/ progestogen or tibolone. The Guideline Development Group recommends that clinicians continue to treat women with a history of endometriosis after surgical menopause with combined oestrogen/progestogen or tibolone at least up to the age of natural menopause.

Reference: European Society of Human Reproduction and Embryology (2013). ESHRE guideline: Management of women with endometriosis.

124. Answer: A.

Explanation: Nonsteroidal anti-inflammatory drugs (NSAIDs) and prostaglandin synthetase inhibitors are the most commonly used drugs for the treatment of dysmenorrhoea. All NSAIDs appear equally effective, although ibuprofen is most often used because it has a low incidence of side effects. Although licensed specifically for dysmenorrhoea, there are concerns that mefenamic acid is more likely to induce seizures in overdose and has a low therapeutic window.

References: Marjoribanks J, Proctor ML, Farquhar C (2010). Nonsteroidal anti-inflammatory drugs for primary dysmenorrhoea. *Cochrane Database System Review* Jan 20 (1), CD001751.
Proctor M, Farquhar C (2006). Diagnosis and management of dysmenorrhoea. *BMJ* 13, 332 (7550), 1134–1138.

125. Answer: C.

Explanation: The clinical presentation of adnexal torsion, like other pathologies, is sometimes with acute onset of pelvic pain but it can also be more nonspecific and frequently presents diagnostic difficulties. Nausea and vomiting are common presenting features occurring in 85% of cases. A recently published scoring system identified five criteria that were independently associated with adnexal torsion and allowed cases to be placed into low-risk and high-risk groups. This patient is unlikely to be pregnant or ovulating given the use of Mirena intrauterine system.

	Criterion	Adjusted odds ratio (95% CI)
1	Unilateral lumbar or abdominal pain	4.1 (1.2–14)
2	Pain duration >8 h	8.0 (1.7–37.5)
3	Vomiting	7.9 (2.3–27)
4	Absence of leucorrhoea/metrorrhagia	12.6 (2.3–67.6)
5	Ovarian cyst >5 cm by ultrasound	10.6 (2.9–38.8)

CI, confidence interval.

Reference: Damigos E, Ptychio I, Johns J, Ross J (2012). An update on the diagnosis and management of ovarian torsion. *The Obstetrician & Gynaecologist* 14 (4), 229–236.

126. Answer: D.

Explanation: The history and examination are highly suggestive of trichomoniasis, although it would be important to assess for other STIs.

Reference: Royal College of Obstetricians and Gynaecologists. StratOG, core training, sexual and reproductive health.

127. Answer: C.

Explanation: Vulvodynia is the term used to describe the sensation of vulval burning and soreness in the absence of any obvious skin condition or infection. The pain is burning and sore in nature; itching is not usually a problem. Vestibulodynia is pain with light touch, e.g. with tampon use or sexual intercourse, and there are usually no symptoms at other times.

References: Vulval Pain Society. Vulvodynia – Vulval Pain Society. 2015. Available from: http://www.vulvalpainsociety.org/vps/index.php/vulval-conditions/vulvodynia. Nagandla K, Sivalingam N (2014). Vulvodynia: Integrating current knowledge into clinical practice. *The Obstetrician & Gynaecologist* 16, 259–267.

128. Answer: B.

Explanation: Etidronate is the only one of the four bisphosphonates listed that has not been shown to reduce hip fractures. All of them reduce the risk of vertebral fracture by reducing osteoclast bone resorption. Only oestrogen has been shown to influence the laying down of new bone. Bisphosphonates are used in conjunction with oral vitamin D and calcium. Regular weight-bearing exercise and avoidance of smoking are also important in the treatment of postmenopausal osteoporosis.

References: Kwun S, Laufgraben MJ, Gopalakrishnan G (2012). Prevention and treatment of postmenopausal osteoporosis. *The Obstetrician & Gynecologist* 14, 251–256.
Wells GA, Cranney A, Peterson J, et al. (2008). Etidronate for the primary and secondary prevention of osteoporotic fractures in postmenopausal women. *Cochrane Database System Review* Jan 23 (1), CD003376.

129. Answer: A.

Explanation: Ultrasound findings are most consistent with a dermoid cyst of the right ovary. Her symptoms and examination suggest ovarian torsion as the source of her pain. The next best step is laparoscopy with detorsion of the ovary; ovarian cystectomy can be performed at that stage or a few weeks later. Observation is not appropriate as time increases the chance of losing the ovary and decreased fecundity. Laparoscopy also allows visualization of the appendix. Magnetic resonance imaging is not necessary because the vaginal ultrasound and her symptoms are consistent with ovarian torsion. Laparotomy should be avoided if possible to minimize adhesive complications.

Reference: Damigos E, Johns J, Ross J. (2012). An update on the diagnosis and management of ovarian torsion. *The Obstetrician & Gynecologist* 14, 229–236.

130. Answer: B.

Explanation: On the day of surgery, dehydration is avoided by reducing the period of 'no oral fluid' to 2 hours for clear fluids. The use of complex carbohydrate drinks in nondiabetic patients has been shown to be beneficial in colorectal surgery, reducing preoperative thirst, hunger and anxiety and postoperative insulin resistance. This reduces length of stay and improves patient experience. Mechanical bowel preparation has time and cost implications and is unpleasant for patients. It is also associated with morbidity, and there is no evidence that it improves the outcome for colorectal patients having elective rectal surgery in which bowel continuity is restored.

Reference: Enhanced Recovery in Gynaecology (2013). Scientific Impact Paper No. 36.

131. Answer: D.

Explanation: For women who have a hysterectomy with ovarian conservation at age 50 to 54, and who are at average risk for ovarian cancer, coronary heart disease, breast cancer and stroke, the probability of surviving to age 80 is 63% (without oestrogen replacement therapy) compared with 54% if oophorectomy is performed (again without oestrogen replacement therapy). This 9% difference in survival is primarily due to fewer women dying of coronary artery disease (7.57% versus 15.95%) and hip fracture (3.38% versus 4.96%) far outweighing the 0.47% mortality rate from ovarian cancer after simple hysterectomy for benign disease. If surgery occurs at ages 55 to 59, the survival advantage is 3.9%. At age 65, there is no significant difference in survival.

Reference: Parker WH, Broder MS, et al. (2005). Ovarian conservation at time of hysterectomy for benign disease. *Obstetrics and Gynecology* 106, 219–226.

132. Answer: B.

Explanation: Second-generation combined oral contraceptive pills do not show any improvement in premenstrual syndrome (PMS) symptoms, because the daily progestogen in the second-generation pills (e.g. levonorgestrel or norethisterone) reproduces PMS-type symptoms. Fluoxetine is associated with a more rapid improvement but, at follow-up, CBT has been associated with better maintenance of treatment effects compared with fluoxetine. Luteal phase and continuous dosing with SSRIs can be recommended, and there are data to suggest that improvement of symptoms with luteal-phase dosing continues into the postmenstrual phase. B_6-related peripheral neuropathy can occur with high doses of B_6 so the daily dose should be limited to 10 mg. Danazol is effective, although its use is limited because of its potential irreversible virilizing effect.

Reference: Royal College of Obstetricians and Gynaecologists (2007). Management Green-top Guideline No. 48. Premenstrual syndrome. London.

133. Answer: A.

Explanation: Antibiotic prophylaxis is not required for laparoscopic surgery unless there are high-risk factors or contaminated wounds.

Reference: Scottish Intercollegiate Guidelines Network (2014). SIGN 104. Antibiotic prophylaxis in surgery, a national clinical guideline.

134. Answer: A.

Explanation: Recurrent candidiasis is defined as four or more episodes of symptomatic candidiasis annually. Treatment regimens in current usage are empirical and are not based on RCTs. Principles of therapy include induction followed by a maintenance regime for 6 months. Cessation of therapy may result in relapse in at least 50% of women.

Reference: van Schalkwyk J, Yudin MH, Allen V et al. (2015). Vulvovaginitis: Screening for and management of trichomoniasis, vulvovaginal candidiasis, and bacterial vaginosis. *Journal of Obstetrics and Gynaecology Canada* 37 (3), 266–274.

135. Answer: C.

Explanation: Congenital adrenal hyperplasia can present with precocious puberty as does McCune–Albright syndrome. Those with complete androgen insensitivity syndrome have a 46XY karyotype.

Reference: Valappil S, Chetan U, Wood N, Gardend A (2012). Mayer–Rokitansky–Küster–Hauser syndrome: Diagnosis and management. *The Obstetrician & Gynaecologist* 14, 93–98.

136. Answer: C.

Explanation: Mature cystic teratomas (dermoids) account for about 15% of all ovarian neoplasms. They tend to be identified in young women, typically around the age of 30 years, and are also the most common ovarian neoplasm in patients younger than 20 years. Uncomplicated ovarian dermoids tend to be asymptomatic and are often discovered incidentally. They do, however, predispose to ovarian torsion, and may then present with acute pelvic pain. They are bilateral in 10% to 15% of cases.

Reference: Outwater EK, Siegelman ES, Hunt JL (2001). Ovarian teratomas: Tumor types and imaging characteristics. *Radiographics* 21 (2), 475–490.

137. Answer: B.

It is generally accepted that CO_2 should be used as a distending medium for diagnostic hysteroscopy only as it is not suitable for operative hysteroscopy or diagnostic procedures; this is in part because blood and endometrial debris collect and obscure the optical field.

Reference: Munro MG, et al. (2012). AAGL Practice Report: Practice Guidelines for the Management of Hysteroscopic Distending Media. *Journal of Minimally Invasive Gynecology* 20 (2), 137–148.

138. Answer: B.

Explanation: Three percent sorbitol is broken down into fructose and glucose; therefore it has an added risk of hyperglycaemia when absorbed in excess.

Reference: Munro MG, et al. (2012). AAGL Practice Report: Practice Guidelines for the Management of Hysteroscopic Distending Media. *Journal of Minimally Invasive Gynecology* 20 (2), 137–148.

139. Answer: A.

Explanation: Lichen planus is a condition that mainly affects the skin by causing an itchy rash. In some cases it affects the mouth, genitals, hair, nails and (rarely) other parts of the body. About half of people with a lichen planus skin rash develop white streaks on the inside of the cheeks, gums or tongue. This is usually painless and not itchy, and may not be noticed unless specifically sought. Lichen planus may occasionally occur in the mouth without any additional skin rash.

Reference: Royal College of Obstetricians and Gynaecologists (2011). Green-top Guideline No. 56. The management of vulval skin disorders. London.

140. Answer: D.

Explanation: The clinical features are suggestive of the late-onset congenital adrenal hyperplasia (clitoromegaly or ambiguous genitalia, precocious pubic hair, excessive growth, hirsutism and oligomenorrhoea). The diagnosis depends on the demonstration of inadequate production of cortisol, aldosterone, or both, in the presence of excess precursor hormones. In 21-hydroxylase deficiency there is a high serum concentration of 17-hydroxyprogesterone and urinary pregnanetriol (a metabolite of 17-hydroxyprogesterone).

Reference: Speiser PW, et al. (2010). Congenital adrenal hyperplasia due to steroid 21-hydroxylase deficiency: An Endocrine Society clinical practice guideline. *The Journal of Clinical Endocrinology and Metabolism* 95 (9), 4133–4160.

141. Answer: B.

Explanation: Both the British National Formulary and the National Institute for Health and Clinical Excellence advise women to consider stopping HRT 4 weeks before elective surgery.

Reference: Royal College of Obstetricians and Gynaecologists (2011). Green-top Guideline No. 19. Venous thromboembolism and hormone replacement therapy, 3rd ed. London.

142. Answer: E.

Explanation: Evidence suggests that transdermal preparations are associated with a lower risk of VTE disease than oral preparations. Universal screening of all women for thrombophilic defects before HRT is difficult to justify, but it is reasonable to screen those with a personal history or strong family history. Even in the presence of a normal thrombophilia screen, a personal history of VTE is usually considered a contraindication to oral HRT, although decisions should be individualized. If it is considered that quality of life is so severely affected that the benefits of HRT outweigh the risks, then a transdermal preparation could be prescribed following a fully informed discussion. The absolute risk of VTE with HRT is low.

References: Royal College of Obstetricians and Gynaecologists (2011). Green-top Guideline No. 19. Venous thromboembolism and hormone replacement therapy, 3rd ed. London.
Bakour SH, Williamson J (2015). Latest evidence on using hormone replacement therapy in the menopause. *The Obstetrician & Gynaecologist* 17, 20–28.

143. Answer: D.

Explanation: Acoustic shadowing is not an indicator of malignancy and is considered a benign finding. The other options are indicators of malignancy, as is an irregular multilocular solid tumour with largest diameter greater than or equal to 100 mm.

Reference: Royal College of Obstetricians and Gynaecologists (2011). Green-top Guideline No. 62. Management of suspected ovarian masses in premenopausal women. London.

144. Answer: D.

Explanation: Girls who have not received any HPV vaccine by the age of 15 will need three doses of the vaccine to have full protection. This is because the response to two doses in older girls is not quite as good as those at the recommended age of 11 to 12 years.

Reference: The human papillomavirus vaccine: Beating cervical cancer – the facts, Public Health England. Available at: https://www.gov.uk/government/publications/the-human-papillomavirus-vaccine-beating-cervical-cancer-the-facts.

145. Answer: C.

Explanation: Following surgery for endometriosis, the postoperative use of a LNG-IUS or the combined hormonal contraceptive for at least 18 to 24 months is recommended for secondary prevention of endometriosis-associated dysmenorrhoea.

Reference: European Society of Human Reproduction and Embryology (2013). ESHRE guideline: Management of women with endometriosis.

146. Answer: E.

Explanation: The finding of an endometrium measuring less than or equal to 5 mm in a woman on HRT reduces the pretest risk of endometrial cancer from 1.0 to 1.5% to 0.1 to 0.2%. An endometrial thickness of 3 mm can be used to exclude endometrial cancer in women who are using continuous combined HRT. It can take up to 6 months for amenorrhoea to develop on continuous combined HRT. Endometrial thickness in patients on sequential HRT, measured soon after withdrawal bleeding, is not significantly different from thickness measured in patients on combined HRT. Patients on HRT with an endometrial thickness of greater than 4 mm could be considered for histologic sampling. The prevalence of abnormal endometrial findings in patients with a thick endometrium is significantly higher than the prevalence observed in patients with unexpected bleeding.

Reference: Otify M, Fuller J, Ross J, Shaikh H, Johns J (2015). Endometrial pathology in the postmenopausal woman – an evidence based approach to management. *The Obstetrician & Gynaecologist* 17, 29–38.

147. Answer: C.

Explanation: Although some tests, such as a hysterosalpingogram (HSG; injection of dye into the uterine cavity followed by an x-ray) or a sonohysterogram (injection of fluid into the uterine cavity while looking with ultrasound) may suggest the presence of intrauterine adhesions, the gold standard is to look directly at the uterine cavity and scar tissue using hysteroscopy.

Reference: Royal College of Obstetricians and Gynaecologists. StratOG, core training, gynaecological problems and early pregnancy loss.

148. Answer: E.

Explanation: Forty percent of women have a variety of symptoms and signs postembolization including diffuse abdominal pain, generalized malaise, anorexia, nausea, vomiting, low-grade fever and leucocytosis. The syndrome is self-limiting and usually resolves within 2 days to 2 weeks. Supportive therapy with intravenous fluids and adequate pain control, including nonsteroidal antiinflammatory drugs, is appropriate.

Reference: Society of Obstetricians and Gynaecologists of Canada (2015). Clinical practice guideline No. 318. The management of uterine leiomyomas. Ottawa.

149. Answer: C.

Explanation: The recommendations include:
- Fluid deficit of 500 ml: ensure that the anaesthetist is aware of the deficit.

- Fluid deficit of 1000 ml: the procedure should be completed as expeditiously as possible. Consider placing Foley catheter in bladder for accurate monitoring of urine output. Consider fluid restriction. Consider intravenous diuretic (e.g. furosemide) administration.
- Fluid deficit of 1500 ml: the procedure should be discontinued. Serum electrolyte values should be obtained and abnormalities managed appropriately. Observe patient for signs of fluid overload and encephalopathy, seizure activity, pulmonary oedema and tachypnoea. Admit for observation and management of complications.

Reference: Society of Obstetricians and Gynaecologists of Canada (2015). Clinical practice guideline No. 322. Endometrial ablation in the management of abnormal uterine bleeding. Ottawa.

Module 14   Subfertility

QUESTIONS

150. Comparing letrozole with clomifene citrate in patients with polycystic ovarian syndrome, clomifene citrate is associated with:

Options

- A. Lower live birth rate.
- B. Lower rate of multiple pregnancy.
- C. Lower incidence of ovarian hyperstimulation.
- D. Better side effects profile.
- E. Higher implantation rate.

151. A 29-year-old with primary subfertility and a BMI of 30 kg/m² is known to have polycystic ovarian syndrome based on anovulation, transvaginal ultrasound appearances of the ovaries and a raised testosterone. She has remained anovulatory despite increasing doses of clomifene citrate over six cycles.

What is the most appropriate next step in her management?

Options

- A. Unstimulated intrauterine insemination.
- B. Continue further three cycles of clomifene citrate.
- C. Continue further six cycles of clomifene citrate.
- D. Gonadotropins.
- E. Metformin.

152. A 25-year-old athlete with a BMI of 18 presents to the fertility clinic after trying for a pregnancy for 2 years. She has oligomenorrhoea and her partner's semen analysis is within the normal range. Her gonadotropin profile shows a low FSH and LH. The oestrogen levels are also low, although the androgen profile is normal.

What is the best strategy for her ovarian stimulation?

Options

   A. Clomifene citrate.
   B. Lifestyle interventions (normalizing weight and exercise) + human menopausal gonadotropins.
   C. Pulsatile GnRH.
   D. Norethisterone 10 mg for 5 to 7 days and clomifene citrate 50 mg on days 2 to 6.
   E. Recombinant FSH + LH preparations.

153. A 36-year-old para 1 is undergoing an IVF cycle. She has egg retrieval and two fresh embryos are transferred. Her initial beta human chorionic gonadotropin is 1600 mIU/ml, and she begins to develop abdominal pain, nausea and vomiting. An ultrasound reveals two gestational sacs and free abdominal fluid. She is not short of breath, her pulse oximetry is 98% on room air and electrolytes and haematocrit and liver function tests are within normal limits.

What grade of ovarian hyperstimulation syndrome should she be categorized as having?

Options

   A. None.
   B. Mild.
   C. Moderate.
   D. Severe.
   E. Critical.

154. A 35-year-old para 0 is in the midst of an IVF cycle. She has undergone egg retrieval following human chorionic gonadotropin administration, and you have just implanted two fresh embryos.

What is the chance that she will develop OHSS?

Options

  A. 5%.
  B. 10%.
  C. 20%.
  D. 30%.
  E. 40%.

155. A patient with subfertility is found to have tubal obstruction following an HSG. There are no known additional pelvic comorbidities (such as PID, previous ectopic pregnancy or endometriosis).

What is the chance that laparoscopy will confirm these findings of occlusion?

Options

  A. 10% of patients.
  B. 25% of patients.
  C. 35% of patients.
  D. 55% of patients.
  E. 65% of patients.

156. A 37-year-old para 0, who has undergone controlled ovarian stimulation for IVF treatment 3 weeks previously, presents with abdominal pain, bloating, nausea and vomiting. She is known to have PCOS and had not ovulated previously with clomifene citrate treatment. She went on to receive antagonist recombinant FSH protocol and was later given human chorionic gonadotropin to trigger ovulation. Ultrasound has shown evidence of ascites with an ovarian size of 14 cm. Her haematocrit was 46%. The patient was admitted to hospital for inpatient treatment.

What is the recommended regime of thromboprophylaxis?

Options

   A. LMWH for the duration of her stay in hospital.
   B. LMWH for the duration of her stay + 5 days after discharge.
   C. LMWH for the duration of her stay + 7 days after discharge.
   D. LMWH for the first 12 weeks of pregnancy.
   E. LMWH until her OHSS symptoms subside.

157. A 39-year-old male presents to a fertility clinic following a repeat semen analysis for oligoasthenoteratozoospermia. The semen analysis results show semen volume (1.0 ml), sperm concentration (2×10^6/ml), total motility (10%), normal forms (1%) and vitality (10%).

What is the appropriate next step in management?

Options

   A. Controlled ovarian stimulation with IUI.
   B. IVF using intracytoplasmic sperm injection technique.
   C. IVF using donor sperm.
   D. Natural cycle IUI.
   E. Testicular biopsy.

158. A male patient presents with history of anosmia, azoospermia, bilateral small testes and gynaecomastia.

What is the best treatment modality?

Options

    A. Bromocriptine.
    B. Clomifene.
    C. Gonadotropins.
    D. Letrozole.
    E. Testosterone replacement.

159. After an IVF cycle and a subsequently positive pregnancy test, a patient develops abdominal pain, nausea, vomiting and mild shortness of breath. Further evaluation reveals normal lung sounds, palpable ascites and a pulse oximetry of 97% on room air. A chest x-ray is normal, the haematocrit is 40% and an ultrasound shows ovaries of 9 cm with evident ascites.

Which of the following is most consistent with severe OHSS?

Options

    A. Shortness of breath.
    B. Haematocrit greater than 40%.
    C. Palpable ascites.
    D. Ovarian size greater than 9 cm.
    E. All of the above.

Module 14 Subfertility

ANSWERS

150. Answer: A.

Explanation: Letrozole is an aromatase inhibitor belonging to the selective oestrogen receptor modulator family. It competitively and reversibly binds the haem component of its cytochrome P450 unit to reduce oestrogen production, but it does not inhibit production of mineralocorticoids or corticosteroids. In those with PCOS, letrozole appears to be associated with a higher live birth rate, lower rate of multiple pregnancy and lower incidence of OHSS compared with treatment with clomifene citrate.

Reference: National Institute for Health and Care Excellence (2015). A summary of selected new evidence relevant to NICE clinical guideline 156. Assessment and treatment for people with fertility problems (2013), evidence update. London.

151. Answer: D.

Explanation: The National Institute for Health and Care Excellence guidelines suggest that treatment with clomifene citrate should not continue for longer than 6 months. For women with World Health Organization Group II ovulation disorders that are known to be resistant to clomifene citrate, one of the following second-line treatments should be considered, depending on clinical circumstances and the woman's preference: laparoscopic ovarian drilling, or combined treatment with clomifene citrate and metformin, or gonadotropins.

Reference: National Institute for Health and Care Excellence (2013). Fertility: Assessment and treatment for people with fertility problems, NICE Clinical Guidelines. London.

152. Answer: B.

Explanation: Women with World Health Organization Group I anovulatory subfertility should be advised that they can improve their chance of regular ovulation, conception and an uncomplicated pregnancy by increasing their body weight if they have a BMI of less than 19 and/or reducing their exercise levels if appropriate. If ovulation induction is required then pulsatile administration of GnRH or gonadotropins with LH activity should be offered.

Reference: National Institute for Health and Care Excellence (2013). Fertility: Assessment and treatment for people with fertility problems, NICE Clinical Guidelines. London.

153. Answer: C.

Explanation: She has developed late-onset OHSS and, because of her twin gestation, she is at greater risk of progressing to a more severe form of OHSS. It is classified as moderate because there is ultrasound evidence of ascites. The course of the condition will typically be longer than with early-onset disease.

Reference: Royal College of Obstetricians and Gynaecologists (2006). Green-top Guideline No. 5. Management of ovarian hyperstimulation syndrome. London.

154. Answer: D.

Explanation: Up to 33% of women undergoing assisted reproductive technology with gonadotropins will develop OHSS. The majority of cases are graded as mild with symptoms including abdominal bloating and discomfort. All women receiving assisted reproductive technology should have a discussion regarding the risks of OHSS and its potential complications. A signed informed consent should also be completed.

Reference: Royal College of Obstetricians and Gynaecologists (2006). Green-top Guideline No. 5. Management of ovarian hyperstimulation syndrome. London.

155. Answer: C.

Explanation: HSG is not a reliable indicator of tubal occlusion but, when it demonstrates that the fallopian tubes are patent, it is very likely that these findings will be confirmed at laparoscopy.

Reference: National Institute for Health and Care Excellence (2013). Fertility: Assessment and treatment for people with fertility problems, NICE Clinical Guidelines. London.

156. Answer: D.

Explanation: Evidence from recent studies suggests that not only does IVF double the risk of VTE compared with natural conception, but the risk in the first trimester is fourfold higher and the risk of PE during the first trimester is seven times higher. Women with OHSS are particularly prone to VTE in the upper body.

Reference: Royal College of Obstetricians and Gynaecologists (2015). Green-top Guideline No. 37a. Reducing the risk of venous thromboembolism during pregnancy and the puerperium. London.

157. Answer: E.

Explanation: Testicular biopsy, which can be achieved by an open or percutaneous needle approach, is useful in severe oligospermia and azoospermia, and can facilitate sperm recovery for ICSI. The disadvantage of proceeding to IVF using the ICSI technique is difficulty in obtaining a male sample on the egg retrieval day. IUI is not suitable for severe oligospermia. IVF using donor sperm is an option, but most couples would prefer an attempt at achieving fertility with parental sperm in the first instance.

Reference: Karavolos S, Stewart J, Evbuomwan I, McEleny K, Aird I (2013). Assessment of the infertile male *The Obstetrician & Gynaecologist* 15, 1–9.

158. Answer: C.

Explanation: This is likely to be Kallmann's syndrome in which the neurons responsible for releasing GnRH fail to migrate to the hypothalamus. Treatment of the associated hypogonadotropic hypogonadism is with gonadotropins or a pulsatile GnRH pump.

Reference: National Institute for Health and Care Excellence (2013). Fertility: Assessment and treatment for people with fertility problems, NICE Clinical Guidelines. London.

159. Answer: C.

Explanation: This patient has severe OHSS based on her palpable abdominal ascites. These patients are usually intravascularly volume depleted, but the haematocrit is not high enough to warrant a diagnosis of 'severe' based on this criterion alone (needs to be greater than 45%). The shortness of breath is most likely caused by abdominal splinting by the ascites. Ovarian size as a criterion for 'severe' would be greater than or equal to 12 cm (using ovarian size in patients who have undergone egg retrieval is considered to be less reliable than preretrieval). Progression to critical OHSS would require the development of tense ascites, large hydrothorax, a haematocrit greater than 55%, WBC greater than 25, oliguria (urine output less than 1 L/day), thromboembolism or the development of adult respiratory distress syndrome.

Reference: Royal College of Obstetricians and Gynaecologists (2006). Green-top Guideline No. 5. Management of ovarian hyperstimulation syndrome. London.

Module 15 Sexual and reproductive health

QUESTIONS

160. A 24-year-old presents to the A&E department with pelvic pain and vaginal discharge. On examination she is found to be pyrexial (38°C) with moderate lower abdominal tenderness. Vaginal examination confirms bilateral adnexal tenderness and cervical motion tenderness.

Which of the following clinical features are not suggestive of PID?

Options

    A. Lower abdominal pain which is typically bilateral.
    B. Deep dyspareunia.
    C. Abnormal vaginal bleeding, including post coital, intermenstrual and menorrhagia.
    D. Abnormal vaginal or cervical discharge which is often purulent.
    E. Lower abdominal pain which is typically unilateral.

161. A 34-year-old woman with a BMI of 29, who has been taking enalapril for essential hypertension, requests the combined oral contraceptive pill. Her BP is well controlled on this treatment and today is 134/88 mm Hg.

To which UK Medical Eligibility Criteria would well-controlled hypertension be considered?

Options

    A. 1.
    B. 2.
    C. 3.
    D. 4.
    E. 5.

162. A 36-year-old para 2 who is HIV positive with a CD4 count of 73 has been recently started on antiretrovirals. She has attended for her routine cervical smear and mentions that she has developed an ulcer on her labia. Clinically this is vulval herpes simplex virus.

What is the best treatment regime?

Options

    A. Oral aciclovir 200 mg five times a day for 5 days.
    B. Oral aciclovir 200 mg 7 to 10 times a day for 5 days.
    C. Oral aciclovir 400 mg five times a day for 5 days.
    D. Oral aciclovir 400 mg five times a day for 7 to 10 days.
    E. Oral aciclovir 800 mg five times a day for 5 days.

163. A 28-year-old nulliparous patient attended for routine cervical screening which has shown borderline changes and HPV inadequate results. She is not currently sexually active and has had normal smear results before this test.

What is the next appropriate step in management?

Options

    A. Refer to colposcopy.
    B. Repeat cytology only in 3 months.
    C. Repeat cytology and HPV in 3 months.
    D. Repeat cytology and HPV in 6 months.
    E. Repeat cytology and HPV in 12 months.

164. An 18-year-old nulliparous patient attends the gynaecology clinic for heavy painful menstrual bleeding. She is in a sexual relationship with a new partner and both have tested negative for STIs, though she has had a previously treated chlamydia infection. She does not want any children in the near future. She takes lamotrigine for epilepsy control and has not suffered any seizures for 3 years. General and pelvic examinations are normal, and her BMI is 30.

What is the best appropriate method of contraception in her situation?

Options

    A. Combined oral contraceptive pill.
    B. Depot medroxyprogesterone acetate.
    C. Evra patch.
    D. Levonorgestrel-releasing intrauterine system.
    E. NuvaRing

165. A 35-year-old nulliparous patient is HIV positive and takes efavirenz and nevirapine. She is using a 30-mcg oestrogen combined oral contraceptive preparation as well as barrier contraception. She finished a pill packet 10 days ago, forgot to restart again and had unprotected sexual intercourse 2 days ago. She also missed two pills in her first week of the previous pill packet. A chlamydia urine polymerase chain reaction test is positive. She attends asking for emergency contraception.

What is the most appropriate method of emergency contraception in this situation?

Options

    A. 1.5 mg levonorgestrel as soon as possible.
    B. 3 mg levonorgestrel as soon as possible.
    C. LNG-IUS as soon as possible.
    D. The copper IUD as soon as possible.
    E. Ulipristal acetate single 30 mg tablet as soon as possible.

166. A 50-year-old para 2 attends the outpatient gynaecology clinic for HRT advice. She has not had a period for 2 years and has been suffering with increasing hot flushes and sweating. She also reports decreased sexual desire. Detailed history, general and pelvic examinations are unremarkable.

What is the most appropriate HRT regime?

Options

    A. Low-dose vaginal oestrogen.
    B. Topical oestrogen preparation.
    C. Combined oestrogen progesterone preparation orally.
    D. Cyclic oestrogen progesterone preparation orally.
    E. Tibolone.

167. A 28-year-old patient is referred from the A&E department with lower abdominal pain and vaginal discharge. On examination she has a temperature of 37.3°C, a pulse of 86 bpm and a BP of 120/83 mm Hg. Her abdomen is slightly tender in the LIF region. On vaginal examination there is a mild corresponding adnexal tenderness, the IUCD threads are seen and a swab of mucopurulent discharge is taken. She mentions that she has a new sexual partner and has not used barrier contraception.

What is the most appropriate next step in her management?

Options

- A. Intravenous PID-targeted antibiotics + IUCD removal immediately.
- B. Oral PID-targeted antibiotics + IUCD removal immediately.
- C. Oral PID-targeted antibiotics and, if no improvement in symptoms, remove IUCD in 24 hours.
- D. Oral PID-targeted antibiotics and, if no improvement in symptoms, remove IUCD in 48 hours.
- E. Oral PID-targeted antibiotics and, if no improvement in symptoms, remove IUCD in 72 hours.

168. A hysteroscopic tubal sterilization using flexible microinserts (Essure) is performed. The procedure time is about 30 minutes (from insertion to removal of hysteroscope), and there was a concern regarding possible perforation due to a sudden loss of resistance at insertion.

What is the suggested method of confirming that the procedure has been successful?

Options

- A. Hysterosalpingogram.
- B. Magnetic resonance imaging.
- C. Transvaginal ultrasound scan.
- D. Pelvic x-ray.
- E. Diagnostic laparoscopy.

Module 15   Sexual and reproductive health

ANSWERS

160. Answer: E.

Explanation: A diagnosis of PID, and empirical antibiotic treatment, should be considered in any young (under 25) sexually active woman who has recent onset bilateral lower abdominal pain associated with local tenderness on bimanual vaginal examination, and in whom pregnancy has been excluded.

Reference: UK National Guideline for the Management of Pelvic Inflammatory Disease (2011). Clinical Effectiveness Group, British Association for Sexual Health and HIV.

161. Answer: C.

Explanation: Medical eligibility criteria (MEC) relate to the safety of contraceptive methods in people with medical conditions. The UKMEC are adapted from World Health Organization Medical Eligibility Criteria (WHOMEC). Well-controlled hypertension is UKMEC Category 3 for combined oral contraception. This means that the risks generally outweigh the benefits, and it should not normally be considered for use unless other more appropriate methods are not available or acceptable. Most other methods of contraception are likely to be suitable for this woman. A UKMEC Category 1 indicates that there is no restriction; Category 2 that this method can be generally used, but more careful follow-up may be required; and, for Category 4, that use poses an unacceptable health risk. Category 5 does not exist.

Reference: UK Medical Eligibility Criteria for contraceptive use and Selected Practice Recommendations, Clinical Guidance, Faculty of Sexual & Reproductive Healthcare. Available from: http://www.fsrh.org/pages/Clinical_Guidance_1.asp.

162. Answer: D.

Explanation: Ideally, all those with HIV and suspected genital herpes should be referred to a specialist in genitourinary medicine for diagnosis, treatment, screening for STIs, counselling regarding risks to themselves and others and follow-up (especially if they are known to have a low CD4 count). Provided that the infection is uncomplicated and not severe, treatment with double the standard dose of antiviral should be considered. Recommended regimes for people with advanced HIV therefore are oral aciclovir 400 mg five times daily for 7 to 10 days, vanciclovir 500 mg to 1 g twice daily for 10 days or famciclovir 250 to 500 mg three times daily for 10 days. In severe cases, intravenous aciclovir may be required. If she has had herpes simplex virus in the past, this presentation could be part of an immune reconstitution inflammatory syndrome after starting antiretrovirals, which could prove difficult to manage.

Reference: British Association for Sexual Health and HIV (2007). National guideline for the management of genital herpes.

163. Answer: D.

Reference: Cervical screening: programme overview. 2015. Available from: https://www .gov.uk/guidance/cervical-screening-programme-overview.

164. Answer: D.

Explanation: Women with a history of epilepsy who are not taking anticonvulsants or are taking antiepileptic drugs that do not induce liver enzymes (for example, gabapentin, levetiracetam, valproate and vigabatrin) can use any hormonal method. If a woman on lamotrigine wishes to use combined hormonal contraception (pill, patch or ring), an increased dose may be required as serum levels of lamotrigine are reduced. For patients who are currently not diagnosed with an active STI, an IUCD can be used and it may be beneficial in managing her heavy painful periods.

References: Faculty of Sexual and Reproductive Healthcare Clinical Effectiveness Unit (2010) Antiepileptic drugs and contraception and the guidance. London.
Faculty of Sexual and Reproductive Healthcare Clinical Guidance (2011). Drug interactions with hormonal contraception. London.

165. Answer: B.

Explanation: The copper IUD can be inserted up to 120 hours (5 days) after unprotected sex. Levonorgestrel can be used within 72 hours (3 days) of unprotected sexual intercourse and for Ulipristal acetate it is 120 hours (5 days). Ulipristal acetate is not recommended in women who are currently taking liver enzyme-inducing drugs or who have taken them within the past 28 days. If an IUD is unsuitable, 3 mg of levonorgestrel can be given as a single dose as soon as possible within 120 hours.

Reference: Faculty of Sexual and Reproductive Healthcare Clinical Guidance (2011). Emergency contraception. London.

166. Answer: E.

Explanation: A systemic preparation will be required to control vasomotor symptoms, and Tibolone is licensed for treating decreased libido.

Reference: Rees M, Stevenson J, Hope S, Rozenberg S, Palacios S (2009). Commission on human medicines (formerly the Committee on Safety of Medicines). In: *Management of the Menopause*, 5th ed. Boca Raton: CRC Press.

167. Answer: E.

Explanation: For women using intrauterine contraception with symptoms and signs suggestive of pelvic infection, appropriate antibiotics should be started. There is no need to remove the IUD in someone who is not unwell unless symptoms fail to resolve within the following 72 hours, or unless the woman wishes removal.

Reference: Faculty of Sexual and Reproductive Healthcare Clinical Guidance (2007). Intrauterine contraception. London.

168. Answer: A.

Explanation: In Europe, the licence for Essure states that transvaginal ultrasound scan (TVUSS), pelvic x-ray or HSG can be used to confirm placement of microinserts. The manufacturer states that pelvic x-ray or TVUSS may be used as the first-line confirmatory test in Europe, but that HSG should be used in the following circumstances:

- There was concern regarding possible perforation due to either excessive force and/or a sudden loss of resistance at insertion.
- There was difficulty identifying the tubal ostia due to anatomic variation or technical factors (e.g. poor distension, suboptimal lighting or endometrial debris). Health-professional uncertainty regarding microinsert placement at insertion.
- Procedure time greater than 15 minutes (from insertion to removal of hysteroscope).
- Microinsert placement with 0 (zero) or greater than eight trailing coils (i.e. coils protruding inside the uterine cavity).
- Unusual postprocedural pain, either transient or persistent, or onset at some later point postprocedure, without any identifiable cause.
- If x-ray or TVUSS is equivocal or unsatisfactory.

Reference: Faculty of Sexual and Reproductive (2014). Male and female sterilisation, summary of recommendations. London.

QUESTIONS

169. A 25-year-old patient is due to undergo laparoscopic management of her ectopic pregnancy, but is questioning whether salpingectomy is essential.

In counselling her about salpingotomy versus salpingectomy, which statement is correct?

Options

A. One in 5 women may need further treatment including methotrexate and/or a salpingectomy.

B. There is a higher risk of surgical complications with salpingotomy versus salpingectomy.

C. The chance of recurrent ectopic is higher if she undergoes salpingectomy.

D. The chance of subsequent intrauterine pregnancy is higher if she undergoes salpingectomy.

E. The risk of needing blood transfusion is higher with salpingotomy.

170. A 41-year-old patient has been diagnosed with gestational trophoblastic neoplasm 6 months after a complete hydatidiform mole. Her pretreatment beta human chorionic gonadotropin (hCG) was 15,000 IU, and a recent computed tomography scan has suggested a possible single lung metastasis.

What is the best modality of treatment?

Options

- A. Intramuscular methotrexate alternating daily with folinic acid for 1 week followed by 6 rest days until the hCG has returned to normal and then for a further 6 consecutive weeks.
- B. Intramuscular methotrexate alternating daily with folinic acid for 1 week followed by 6 rest days until the hCG has returned to normal, and then for a further 6 consecutive months.
- C. Intravenous methotrexate alternating daily with folinic acid for 1 week followed by 6 rest days until the hCG has returned to normal, and then for a further 6 months.
- D. Intravenous multiagent chemotherapy, which includes combinations of methotrexate, dactinomycin, etoposide, cyclophosphamide and vincristine until hCG level has returned to normal.
- E. Intravenous multiagent chemotherapy, which includes combinations of methotrexate, dactinomycin, etoposide, cyclophosphamide and vincristine until the hCG has returned to normal and then for a further 6 consecutive weeks.

171. A 28-year-old patient attends an early pregnancy unit for a reassurance scan at 8 weeks' gestation. Transvaginal views show a mean sac diameter of 3.5 cm and a CRL of 10 mm with no visible heartbeat. The internal os appears closed on scan and there is no vaginal bleeding.

What are the scan findings likely to suggest?

Options

- A. Early pregnancy demise.
- B. Incomplete miscarriage.
- C. Inevitable miscarriage.
- D. Normal ongoing intrauterine pregnancy.
- E. Pregnancy of indeterminate viability.

172. A 28-year-old woman is admitted with severe right-sided lower abdominal pain. Her pulse is 90 bpm with a BP of 110/70 mm Hg and a transvaginal ultrasound scan shows a 2.5 cm complex right adnexal mass. There is colour flow on Doppler but no free fluid in the pouch of Douglas. A pregnancy test is positive with beta hCG of 1400 IU/L, and there is no evidence of an intrauterine pregnancy. The serum progesterone is 24 nmol/L.

What is the most appropriate next step in her management?

Options

    A. Diagnostic laparoscopy with or without surgery.
    B. Expectant inpatient management.
    C. Expectant outpatient management.
    D. Intramuscular methotrexate injection.
    E. Computed tomographic scan of the pelvis.

173. A 20-year-old para 0 attends for an early pregnancy scan at 12 weeks. An embryo with a CRL of 20 mm is identified with no fetal heart action seen. She opts for medical management.

What is the appropriate next step in management?

Options

    A. Mifepristone followed 12 hours later by misoprostol 400 mcg.
    B. Mifepristone followed 24 hours later by misoprostol 800 mcg.
    C. Mifepristone followed 36 hours later by misoprostol 800 mcg.
    D. Misoprostol 400 mcg.
    E. Misoprostol 1200 mcg.

174. A 29-year-old patient presents with abdominal distension and vaginal bleeding at 12 weeks' gestation. A transvaginal ultrasound scan suggests a molar pregnancy with bilateral enlarged multicystic ovaries. The cysts are thin walled and have clear contents. There is no obvious free fluid in the pelvis.

What is the most likely diagnosis?

Options

- A. Mucinous cystadenoma.
- B. Ovarian cystadenofibroma.
- C. Serous cystadenoma.
- D. Struma ovarri.
- E. Theca lutein cyst.

175. In a patient with recurrent miscarriage, the diagnosis of antiphospholipid syndrome requires:

Options

- A. Lupus anticoagulant (LA) present in plasma, on two or more occasions at least 6 weeks apart.
- B. Anticardiolipin (aCL) antibody of immunoglobulin G (IgG) and/or IgM isotype in serum or plasma, present in low titre, on two occasions, at least 12 weeks apart.
- C. aCL antibody of IgG and/or IgM isotype in serum or plasma, present in less than 40 GPL units or MPL units, on two occasions, at least 12 weeks apart.
- D. Anti-b2–glycoprotein I antibody of IgG and/or IgM isotype in serum or plasma (less than the 99th centile on titre), present on two occasions at least 12 weeks apart.
- E. Anti-b2–glycoprotein I antibody of IgG and/or IgM isotype in serum or plasma (greater than the 99th centile on titre), present on two occasions at least 12 weeks apart.

ANSWERS

169. Answer: A.

Explanation: The proportion of women with a subsequent intrauterine pregnancy is significantly lower in patients who undergo a salpingectomy compared with women who have a salpingotomy. There is no statistically significant difference in the need for a blood transfusion between the two, nor is there a difference in the incidence of surgical complications between both groups. There is, however, a significant increase in the need for further intervention in those who have a salpingotomy compared with salpingectomy.

Reference: National Institute for Health and Care Excellence (2012). National guideline: Ectopic pregnancy and miscarriage: Diagnosis and initial management in early pregnancy of ectopic pregnancy and miscarriage. National Collaborating Centre for Women's and Children's Health.

170. Answer: A.

Explanation: The need for chemotherapy following a complete mole is 15% and 0.5% after a partial mole. Using the Federation of Gynaecology and Obstetrics 2000 scoring system: those with scores less than or equal to 6 are at low risk and are treated with single-agent intramuscular methotrexate alternating daily with folinic acid for 1 week followed by 6 rest days; those with scores greater than or equal to 7 are at high risk and are treated with intravenous multiagent chemotherapy, which includes combinations of methotrexate, dactinomycin, etoposide, cyclophosphamide and vincristine.

Treatment is continued in all cases until the hCG level has returned to normal and then for a further 6 consecutive weeks. The cure rate for women with a score less than or equal to 6 is almost 100%; the rate for women with a score greater than or equal to 7 is 95%.

Reference: Royal College of Obstetricians and Gynaecologists (2010). Green-top Guideline No. 38. The management of gestational trophoblastic disease. London.

171. Answer: A.

Explanation: The CRL is 10 mm, which means that embryonic cardiac activity should be seen using a transvaginal scan at this stage. This is likely to represent a missed miscarriage, and the National Institute for Health and Care Excellence guideline advice is that if the CRL is 7.0 mm or more with transvaginal scanning and there is no visible cardiac activity, then a second confirmatory opinion should be sought or a repeat scan arranged after a minimum of 7 days before making a firm diagnosis.

Reference: National Institute for Health and Care Excellence (2012). National guideline: Ectopic pregnancy and miscarriage: Diagnosis and initial management in early pregnancy of ectopic pregnancy and miscarriage. National Collaborating Centre for Women's and Children's Health.

172. Answer: A.

Explanation: The most likely diagnosis is ectopic pregnancy. The scan did not confirm or exclude this, and the right-sided mass could represent a corpus luteum. Beta hCG levels are borderline for transvaginal ultrasound scan visualization of an intrauterine pregnancy. Serum progesterone levels are also not helpful in differentiating between a thriving and a failing pregnancy. In this situation, if the patient is haemodynamically stable, a repeat blood test to establish a trend would not be inappropriate, but the severity of the pain would favour performing a diagnostic laparoscopy to diagnose or exclude ectopic pregnancy with a small risk of negative laparoscopy. Methotrexate is not ideal unless a confirmation of ectopic pregnancy is seen.

Reference: Kirk E, Bottomley C, Bourne T (2013). Diagnosing ectopic pregnancy and current concepts in the management of pregnancy of unknown location. *Human Reproduction Update* 20 (2), 250–261.

173. Answer: D.

Explanation: Mifepristone is no longer recommended for missed or incomplete miscarriage. Vaginal misoprostol is advised, but oral therapy is an alternative if preferred. In outpatient management of miscarriage, a 400 mcg dose of vaginal misoprostol appears to be as effective at inducing complete miscarriage as an 800 mcg dose, and is associated with a reduced rate of fever and rigors, and improved patient satisfaction.

Reference: National Institute for Health and Care Excellence (2012). National guideline: Ectopic pregnancy and miscarriage: Diagnosis and initial management in early pregnancy of ectopic pregnancy and miscarriage. National Collaborating Centre for Women's and Children's Health.

174. Answer: E.

Explanation: Theca lutein cysts are thought to occur with excessive circulating gonadotropins such as beta hCG. Hyperplasia of the theca interna cells is the predominant characteristic on histology. The ovarian parenchyma is often markedly oedematous and frequently contains foci of luteinized stromal cells.

References: Montz FJ, Schlaerth JB, Morrow CP (1988). The natural history of theca lutein cysts. *Obstetrics and Gynecology* 72 (2), 247–251.
Royal College of Obstetricians and Gynaecologists (2010). Green-top Guideline No. 38. The management of gestational trophoblastic disease. London.

175. Answer: E.

Explanation: To diagnose antiphospholipid syndrome the patient must have at least one of the clinical criteria and one of the laboratory criteria listed next:
Clinical:

- One or more unexplained deaths of morphologically normal fetus at or beyond the 10th week of gestation.
- One or more preterm births of a morphologically normal neonate before the 34th week of gestation because of (1) eclampsia or (2) recognized features of placental insufficiency.

- Three or more unexplained consecutive spontaneous miscarriages before the 10th week of gestation, with maternal anatomic or hormonal abnormalities and paternal and maternal chromosomal causes excluded.

Laboratory criteria:

- Lupus anticoagulant present in plasma on two or more occasions at least 12 weeks apart.
- Anticardiolipin antibody of IgG and/or IgM isotype in serum or plasma, present in medium or high titre (i.e., greater than 40 GPL units or MPL units, or greater than the 99th centile), on two or more occasions, at least 12 weeks apart.
- Anti-b2–glycoprotein I antibody of IgG and/or IgM isotype in serum or plasma (greater than the 99th centile on titre), present on two or more occasions at least 12 weeks apart.

Reference: Keeling D, Mackie I, Moore GW, Greer IA, Greaves M, British Committee for Standards in Haematology (2012). Guidelines on the investigation and management of antiphospholipid syndrome. *British Journal of Haemotology* 157 (1), 47–58.

QUESTIONS

176. A 55-year-old patient has had a colposcopic examination for a suspicious well-circumscribed vulval lesion and vulvar intraepithelial neoplasia 3 is identified at histopathology.

What is the most appropriate next step in management?

Options

    A. 5-Fluorouracil cream.

    B. Imiquimod cream 5%.

    C. Local excision.

    D. Local destruction by laser.

    E. Vulvectomy.

177. A 65-year-old patient undergoes a TAH+BSO for a suspicious 8-cm right ovarian mass and normal CA-125. She had originally presented with postmenopausal bleeding. Frozen section examination demonstrates Call–Exner bodies.

It is likely that the pathology specimen will also demonstrate which of the following?

Options

    A. Brenner cell tumour.

    B. Clear cell carcinoma of the cervix.

    C. Endometrial hyperplasia.

    D. Mucinous ovarian carcinoma.

    E. Serous adenocarcinoma.

178. In counselling a patient who had recently tested positive for BRCA1 mutation, risk-reducing bilateral salpingo-oophorectomy (RRBSO) decreases ovarian cancer risk by:

Options

    A. 30 to 45%.
    B. 50 to 55%.
    C. 60 to 75%.
    D. 80 to 95%.
    E. 100%.

179. A 25-year-old para 0, who wished to preserve future fertility, underwent a cervical conization after an unsatisfactory colposcopy. The conization specimen demonstrated an invasive carcinoma of the cervix infiltrating 2.5 mm below the basement membrane. There was no evidence of lymphovascular space involvement, and the margins of the cone were free of dysplasia or carcinoma.

What would be the best strategy of management for this patient?

Options

    A. External beam radiotherapy.
    B. External beam radiotherapy followed by brachytherapy.
    C. No further therapy.
    D. Radical hysterectomy.
    E. Simple hysterectomy.

180. A 45-year-old patient is found to have a large cervical cancer infiltrating into the right parametrium. Rectovaginal examination suggests parametrial involvement, although not reaching the pelvic sidewall. A chest x-ray and cystoscopy were both clear. A computed tomography of the abdomen and pelvis, however, shows an enlarged, suspicious left paraaortic lymph node.

What stage of disease is this?

Options

    A. Stage IIA.
    B. Stage IIB.
    C. Stage IIIB.
    D. Stage IVA.
    E. Stage IVB.

181. A 29-year-old patient is found to have high-grade squamous dyskaryosis at routine cervical smear at 7 weeks' gestation. Colposcopic biopsies show early invasive disease. A subsequent cold-knife conization at 17 weeks shows microinvasive carcinoma of the cervix with clear surgical margins.

What would be the most appropriate plan of action?

Options

    A. Caesarean section at 34 weeks followed by radical hysterectomy.
    B. Caesarean section at 34 weeks followed by simple hysterectomy.
    C. Radical hysterectomy before 20 weeks of gestation.
    D. Induction of labour at 34 weeks aiming for vaginal delivery.
    E. Vaginal delivery at term, providing there are no obstetric contraindications.

182. A 60-year-old patient who had previously had a TAH+BSO for benign disease is found to have an exophytic 1-cm nodule in the upper part of the vagina. Biopsies obtained demonstrate an adenocarcinoma.

What is the most likely diagnosis?

Options

- A. Primary vaginal cancer.
- B. DES-associated clear cell adenocarcinoma.
- C. Metastasis.
- D. Paget's cells are most likely present upon review of the microscopic pathology slides.
- E. Previous gynaecologic cancer was missed at the time of TAH+BSO.

183. In cases of cervical cancer, radical hysterectomy with bilateral pelvic lymphadenectomy can potentially be used to treat all of the following stages of cervical cancer except:

Options

- A. Stage IA1 disease.
- B. Stage IA2 disease with lymphovascular space involvement.
- C. Stage IB1 disease.
- D. Stage IIA disease.
- E. Stage IIB disease.

184. A 47-year-old patient with a history of severe endometriosis is found to have a left-sided, 10-cm unilocular cystic mass with a solid component arising from its wall. A computed tomography scan supports this finding and the CA-125 is 300 U/ml.

These findings raise suspicion of:

Options

- A. Clear cell carcinoma.
- B. Mucinous cystadenoma.
- C. Mucinous cystadenocarcinoma.
- D. Serous cystadenoma.
- E. Granulosa cell tumour.

185. A 55-year-old patient who has a BMI of 39 is scheduled to have a TAH+BSO and pelvic lymphadenectomy for endometrial cancer.

What is the best method to reduce her venous thromboembolic risk?

Options

- A. Antiembolism stockings (thigh or knee length) at admission plus LMWH for 7 days postoperatively.
- B. Antiembolism stockings (thigh or knee length) at admission plus LMWH for 10 days postoperatively.
- C. Antiembolism stockings (thigh or knee length) at admission plus LMWH for 21 days postoperatively.
- D. Intermittent pneumatic compression devices at admission plus LMWH for 14 days postoperatively.
- E. Foot impulse devices at admission plus LMWH for 28 days postoperatively.

186. A 40-year-old patient has had a cervical smear showing moderate/severe dyskaryosis. Colposcopic examination and biopsy confirm CIN II, and she opts for TAH as her family is complete. Histopathology confirms completely excised CIN.

What is the most appropriate follow-up?

Options

- A. No cytology follow-up required.
- B. Vault smear 6 and 12 months after treatment.
- C. Vault smear 6 and 18 months after treatment.
- D. Vault smear 3, 6 and 12 months after treatment.
- E. Vault smear annually for 9 years.

187. In counselling a 45-year-old woman has recently been diagnosed with Stage II cervical squamous carcinoma.

It is reasonable to quote a 5-year survival rate of around:

Options

- A. 30%.
- B. 50%.
- C. 70%.
- D. 90%.
- E. 95%.

188. A 66-year-old patient presented with vulval pruritus. On examination there was a 1.5-cm lesion on her right labia majora with an irregular border; the lesion was tender to touch. An excision biopsy was obtained which showed squamous cell carcinoma with positive margins and invasive disease to 0.8 mm.

What is the most appropriate next step in management?

Options

    A. Chemotherapy.
    B. Radiotherapy.
    C. Right hemivulvectomy with ipsilateral groin lymphadenectomy.
    D. Wide local excision.
    E. Wide local excision plus sentinel lymph node biopsy.

189. A 60-year-old patient presents with a 3-month history of intermittent vaginal bleeding. She has been menopausal since the age of 55 and is otherwise fit and well. The vaginal bleeding was sudden in onset and heavy, with the passage of blood clots and intermittent lower abdominal pain. She has no history of postcoital or contact bleeding, weight loss or anorexia and she was not on HRT. A transvaginal ultrasound scan shows an endometrial thickness of 15 mm and Pipelle biopsy confirms endometrial adenocarcinoma. At TAH+BSO, the left ovary was noted to contain solid tumour.

What is the most likely diagnosis?

Options

    A. Adult granulosa cell tumour.
    B. Dysgerminoma.
    C. Embryonal cell carcinoma.
    D. Endodermal sinus tumour.
    E. Mucinous cystadenoma.

190. A 15-year-old patient presents with left lower abdominal pain. Transvaginal and transabdominal ultrasound scans show a 10-cm solid ovarian mass. The lactate dehydrogenase is elevated with a normal alpha fetoprotein and human chorionic gonadotropin.

What is the most likely diagnosis?

Options

    A. Dysgerminoma.
    B. Embryonal cell carcinoma.
    C. Mucinous cystadenocarcinoma.
    D. Serous cystadenocarcinoma.
    E. Yolk sac tumour.

191. An endometrial Pipelle biopsy result that you have performed a week ago has shown endometrial hyperplasia with atypia. The patient is a 55-year-old para 0 who has a previous history of breast cancer.

When counselling the patient, what would be the chance of her also having an endometrial cancer, if a hysterectomy is performed in the next few weeks?

Options

    A. 1%.
    B. 5%.
    C. 10%.
    D. 25%.
    E. 40%.

192. A 56-year-old patient has had an ultrasound scan, which shows a right adnexal unilocular cystic mass, and subsequent computed tomography scan which has confirmed the same findings but with evidence of peritoneal deposits. Her CA-125 is 10 and the RMI is 30.

Where should she receive her treatment?

Options

    A. Gynaecology unit.
    B. Gynaecology unit with lead gynaecologic oncologist.
    C. Gynaecologic department with interested gynaecologist.
    D. Gynaecologic cancer centre.
    E. Gynaecologic research unit.

ANSWERS

176. Answer: C.

Explanation: Local excision is the treatment of choice for small well-circumscribed lesions, as it has the lowest rate of recurrence. Local destruction by laser is an option, but there are only anecdotal reports of this method. Partial and complete clinical and histologic regression has been shown in small studies with Imiquimod cream 5%, but treatment is limited by side effects and only short-term follow-up data are available; it is also an unlicensed indication. Vulvectomy has been effective, but recurrence may still occur, and function and cosmesis may be impaired. 5-Fluorouracil cream may lead to resolution of some lesions, but results are variable and side effects common; this too is an unlicensed indication.

Reference: Clinical Effectiveness Group, British Association Sexual Health and HIV (2007). UK National Guideline on the Management of Vulval Conditions.

177. Answer: C.

Explanation: Call–Exner bodies are found in adult granulosa cell tumours. Such tumours often produce unopposed oestrogens, which may lead to endometrial hyperplasia or an endometrial adenocarcinoma.

Reference: Ioffe OB, Simsir A, Silverberg SG (2005). Pathology. In: *Practical Gynecologic Oncology*, Berek JS, Hacker NF (Eds.). Philadelphia: Lippincott, Williams and Wilkins.

178. Answer: D.

Explanation: The mainstay of management for women who carry a constitutional BRCA1 or BRCA2 mutation is RRBSO, which reduces the chance of ovarian cancer by 80% to 96% for BRCA1 and BRCA2 carriers. In BRCA1 mutation carriers the risk of breast cancer may also decrease by as much as 56% and for women with a BRCA2 mutation by up to 46%. There remains a residual 1% to 6% risk of primary peritoneal cancer; however, that appears to persist for up to 20 years after oophorectomy.

Reference: Royal College of Obstetricians and Gynaecologists (2015). Scientific Impact Paper No. 48. Management of women with a genetic predisposition to gynaecological cancers. London.

179. Answer: C.

Explanation: Patients with a cervical cancer with less than 3 mm of invasion and absence of lymphovascular space invasion may be treated with simple, extrafascial hysterectomy without lymph node dissection. Therapeutic conization is adequate, however, in those patients wishing to conserve their fertility providing that the surgical margins obtained at the conization are free of disease.

Reference: Krivak TC, McBroom JW, Elkas JC (2011). Cervical and vaginal cancer. In: *Berek & Novak's Gynecology*, Berek JS (Ed.), 15th ed. Philadelphia: Lippincott, Williams and Wilkins, Philadelphia.

180. Answer: B.

Explanation: Cervical cancer is clinically staged. Clinical staging is based on clinical examination, cystoscopy, proctoscopy and chest x-ray findings. The findings at magnetic resonance imaging/computed tomography scanning, laparoscopy etc. may be of value in treatment planning, but do not enter into the determination of clinical stage.

Reference: Stage information for cervical cancer. National Cancer Institute. Cervical Cancer Treatment. 2015. Available from: http://www.cancer.gov/types/cervical/hp/cervical-treatment-pdq.

181. Answer: E.

Explanation: This is Stage IA disease. Evidence suggests that the choice of treatment for cervical cancer diagnosed during pregnancy should be decided in the same manner as for nonpregnant patients. For pregnant women with early stage disease (International Federation of Gynaecology and Obstetrics IA1, IA2, IB) diagnosed after 16 weeks of gestation, treatment may be delayed to allow fetal maturity to occur.

Reference: Scottish Intercollegiate Guidelines Network (2008). Management of cervical cancer, a national clinical guideline.

182. Answer: C.

Explanation: Most vaginal cancers are squamous, not adenocarcinomas. DES-associated, clear cell cancers usually occur after the age of 14 with a peak age at diagnosis around 19 years. This is, therefore, unlikely to be a primary vaginal cancer or a DES-associated adenocarcinoma. Paget's cells are characteristic of breast cancer and indicate only the possible presence of an underlying adenocarcinoma. Given the age of the patient and the tumour histology, a metastatic lesion is most likely.

Reference: Vaginal cancer treatment. National Cancer Institute. Vaginal Cancer Treatment. 2015. Available from: http://www.cancer.gov/types/vaginal/patient/vaginal-treatment-pdq.

183. Answer: E.

Explanation: The approach for Stage IIB and more advanced cancers of the cervix is radiotherapy; chemotherapy may also be given during the course of external beam radiation.

Reference: Cervical cancer treatment, treatment by stage. National Cancer Institute, National Institutes of Health. 2015. Available at: http://www.cancer.gov/types/cervical/hp/cervical-treatment-pdq.

184. Answer: A.

Explanation: Women with endometriosis have a very small chance of developing clear cell or endometrioid types of epithelial ovarian cancer. Around 25% of these types of cancer are thought to arise from endometriosis, and there may be an association with an ARID1A gene mutation.

Reference: Nissenblatt M (2011). Endometriosis-associated ovarian carcinomas. *New England Journal of Medicine* 364 (5), 482–483.

185. Answer: E.

Explanation: VTE prophylaxis should be offered to patients undergoing gynaecologic surgery who are assessed to be at increased risk of VTE. Mechanical VTE prophylaxis should be started at admission choosing antiembolism stockings (thigh or knee length), foot impulse devices or intermittent pneumatic compression devices (again, thigh or knee length). Mechanical VTE prophylaxis should be continued until the patient no longer has significantly reduced mobility.

Pharmacologic VTE prophylaxis should be added for patients who have a low risk of major bleeding, taking into account individual patient factors and according to clinical judgment. This should be continued until the patient no longer has significantly reduced mobility (generally 5–7 days) but should be extended to 28 days postoperatively for patients who have had major cancer surgery in the abdomen or pelvis.

Reference: Treasure T, Hill J (2010). NICE guidance on reducing the risk of venous thromboembolism in patients admitted to hospital. *Journal of the Royal Society of Medicine* 103 (6), 210–212.

186. Answer: C.

Explanation: Women who have had a hysterectomy with CIN present are at potential risk of developing vaginal intraepithelial neoplasia and invasive vaginal disease. There is no clear evidence that colposcopy increases the detection of disease on follow-up. Expert consensus opinion recommends that women who undergo hysterectomy and have completely excised CIN should have vaginal vault cytology at 6 and 18 months after their hysterectomy.

Reference: Guidelines for the NHS Cervical Screening Programme (2010). Colposcopy and programme management, 2nd ed. NHSCSP Publication No. 20.

187. Answer: B.

Explanation: Five-year relative survival ranges from 96% with Stage I disease to 5% at Stage IV. Stage II disease at diagnosis has a 5-year survival rate of 54%. Because survival statistics have a wide standard deviation they cannot be used to predict exactly what will happen to any individual patient.

Reference: National Cancer Institute. Cancer of the Cervix Uteri: SEER Stat Fact Sheets. 2015. Available from: http://seer.cancer.gov/statfacts/html/cervix.html.

188. Answer: D.

Explanation: Lesions less than 2 cm in diameter and confined to the vulva or perineum, with stromal invasion less than or equal to 1.0 mm (International Federation of Gynaecology and Obstetrics Stage IA), can be managed by wide local excision without groin node dissection as the chance of lymph node metastases is very small.

Reference: Royal College of Obstetricians and Gynaecologists (2014). Guidelines for the diagnosis and management of vulval carcinoma. London.

189. Answer: A.

Explanation: Adult granulosa cell tumour is considered to be the most common malignant sex cord ovarian tumour, although it only accounts for 2% to 3% of all ovarian tumours. Patients may present with nonspecific symptoms such as abdominal pain, distension or bloating. In a majority of cases there may be hormonal manifestations caused by oestrogen activity of the tumour. The tumour is associated with endometrial hyperplasia, endometrial polyps and endometrial carcinoma (associated in 3–25% of cases).

Reference: Shah SP, Kobel M, Senz J, Morin RD, Clarke BA, Wiegand KC (2009). Mutation of FOXL2 in granulosa-cell tumors of the ovary. *New England Journal of Medicine* 360 (26), 2719–2729.

190. Answer: A.

Explanation: The three major types of ovarian tumours are epithelial, sex cord and germ cell. Epithelial cell tumours represent the majority of all ovarian neoplasms (approximately 80%). GCTs are rare, comprising less than 20% of all ovarian tumours, with over 95% of them being benign. One form of GCT is a dysgerminoma; it is usually malignant and most commonly affects women of reproductive age. They have been associated with elevations in lactate dehydrogenase, and may occasionally become infiltrated with syncytiotrophoblastic giant cells which produce beta human chorionic gonadotropin. Elevations in alpha-fetoprotein are less common. Preoperative evaluation of all of these markers, including inhibin, is suggested in patients with suspected ovarian GCTs/dysgerminomas.

Reference: Weinberg LE, Lurain JR, Singh DK, Schink JC (2011). Survival and reproductive outcomes in women treated for malignant ovarian germ cell tumors. *Gynecology and Oncology* 121 (2), 285–289.

191. Answer: E.

Explanation: In patients with atypical endometrial hyperplasia there is a risk of progression to endometrial carcinoma, as well as a risk that the patient will actually have an endometrial cancer at hysterectomy. In patients with an endometrial hyperplasia diagnosed by biopsy or curettage, about 40% were found to have a cancer at hysterectomy.

References: Lurain JR (2002). Uterine cancer. In: *Novak's Gynecology*, Berek JS (Ed.), 20th ed. Philadelphia: Lippincott, Williams and Wilkins, p. 1145.
ACOG Practice Bulletin (2005). Management of endometrial cancer. *Obstetrics and Gynecology* 106 (413), 414–415.
Trimble CL, Kauderer J, Zaino R, et al. (2006). Concurrent endometrial carcinoma in women with a biopsy diagnosis of atypical endometrial hyperplasia: A Gynecologic Oncology Group study. *Cancer* 106 (4), 812–819.

192. Answer: D.

Explanation: Although the patient RMI places her in the low-risk group, the presence of peritoneal deposits makes the diagnosis of cancer much more likely. The RMI score is a way of triaging women with suspected ovarian cancer into those who are at low, moderate or high risk of malignancy and that may be managed by a general gynaecologist, or in a cancer unit or cancer centre, respectively. Using a cut-off point for the RMI of 250, a sensitivity of 70% and specificity of 90% can be achieved for identifying cancer, allowing the majority of women with ovarian cancer to be dealt with by gynaecologic oncologists. The RMI would not, however, take account of the computed tomography scan findings and referral to a gynaecologic oncologist is appropriate.

Reference: Royal College of Obstetricians and Gynaecologists (2010). Green-top Guideline No. 34. Ovarian cysts in postmenopausal women. London.

Module 18 Urogynaecology and pelvic floor disorders

QUESTIONS

193. You see a 62-year-old woman in your gynaecology clinic. She presents with urgency, daytime frequency, nocturia and urge leakage.

What is your initial step in management?

Options

    A. Ultrasound examination of pelvis.
    B. Frequency-volume chart.
    C. Urodynamics.
    D. Cystoscopy.
    E. Q-tip test.

194. You see a 52-year-old woman in your urodynamics clinic. The uroflowmetry curve is bell shaped with a maximum flow rate (Q_{max}) of 23 ml/s. The postvoid residual is 50 ml, and multichannel cystometry shows involuntary detrusor contractions during the filling phase which are provoked by the sound of running tap water. The maximum cystometric capacity is 450 ml.

What is the most appropriate diagnosis?

Options

    A. Normal bladder capacity, detrusor overactivity and no voiding dysfunction.
    B. Normal bladder capacity, detrusor overactivity and voiding dysfunction.
    C. Reduced bladder capacity, detrusor overactivity and no voiding dysfunction.
    D. Reduced bladder capacity, detrusor overactivity and voiding dysfunction.
    E. Normal urodynamic studies.

195. You see a 54-year-old para 3 in your gynaecology clinic who presents with a 9-month history of urinary leakage with both exercise and coughing. There is no urgency or frequency, and she is otherwise well with no previous pelvic surgery. On examination she has a BMI of 24 kg/m^2. There is evidence of urine leakage on cough and a grade 1 cystocele.

What is your first-line treatment?

Options

A. Electrical stimulation in combination with pelvic floor muscle training.
B. Pelvic floor muscle training.
C. Duloxetine.
D. Systemic HRT.
E. Tension-free vaginal tape.

196. You see a 60-year-old para 4 in your gynaecology clinic who presents with a 12-month history of urine leakage with exercise and associated urgency. She reports some improvement of the urgency and urge incontinence on oxybutynin. She is otherwise well and has no previous pelvic surgery. Urodynamic studies show detrusor overactivity, urodynamic stress incontinence, normal cystometric capacity and no voiding dysfunction. She is keen for surgical management.

Which of the following describes her risk of worsening of urge symptoms following synthetic midurethral tape?

Options

A. 0.25%.
B. 2.5%.
C. 5%.
D. 25%.
E. 50%.

197. You see a 58-year-old para 4 in your gynaecology clinic for her follow-up appointment. She gives a 10-month history of frequency, urgency and nocturia. She tells you that conservative management, including two antimuscarinic drugs and mirabegron, has not worked adequately.

What intervention would you offer her next?

Options

- A. Transcutaneous tibial nerve stimulation.
- B. Transcutaneous sacral nerve stimulation.
- C. Multicomponent behavioural therapy.
- D. Bladder wall injection with botulinum toxin A.
- E. Bladder wall injection with botulinum toxin B.

198. A 62-year-old woman undergoes surgical treatment for stress urinary incontinence using synthetic midurethral tape.

Which approach and synthetic tape will you use?

Options

- A. Top-down retropubic approach using type 1 macroporous polypropylene tape.
- B. Top-down retropubic approach using type 1 microporous polypropylene tape.
- C. Bottom-up retropubic approach using type 1 macroporous polypropylene tape.
- D. Bottom-up retropubic approach using type 1 microporous polytetrafluoroethylene tape.
- E. Bottom-up retropubic approach using type 1 macroporous polytetrafluoroethylene tape.

199. You see a 63-year-old who presents with stress urinary incontinence. She has completed a 3-month trial of supervised pelvic floor exercises with no improvement but does not wish invasive intervention.

Which pharmacologic agent would it be the most appropriate to offer?

Options

  A. Imipramine.
  B. Desmopressin.
  C. Tolterodine.
  D. Darifenacin.
  E. Duloxetine.

200. You see a 45-year-old patient with multiple sclerosis in your urogynaecology clinic. She is diagnosed with neurogenic stress incontinence.

Which of the following incontinence procedures would be the most suitable to offer?

Options

  A. Autologous fascial sling.
  B. Synthetic retropubic midurethral sling using bottom-top approach.
  C. Synthetic retropubic midurethral sling using top-down approach.
  D. Synthetic transobturator midurethral sling.
  E. Synthetic midurethral single-incision minisling.

201. A 55-year-old para 2 presents with increasing pelvic pressure and a lump in the vagina. She is sexually active. On examination the cervix is found to be at 2 cm beyond the hymen on coughing, and she undergoes a vaginal hysterectomy.

Which of the following is a recommended measure to prevent enterocele formation?

Options

  A. Posterior repair.
  B. Routine sacrospinous fixation.
  C. McCall's culdoplasty.
  D. Moschowitz culdoplasty.
  E. Simple closure of peritoneum.

202. You see a frail 85-year-old woman in your gynaecology clinic. She is known to have vaginal vault prolapse following a vaginal hysterectomy 15 years ago. She has been using a shelf pessary for the management of her prolapse, but she is now keen to seek surgery.

Which of the following is the most appropriate and least invasive procedure that you will offer her?

Options

    A. Posterior repair.
    B. Sacrospinous fixation.
    C. McCall's culdoplasty.
    D. Moschowitz culdoplasty.
    E. Colpocleisis.

203. Your senior house officer asks you to explain the POP-Q system for assessment of prolapse.

Which of the following points and measurements is not part of the POP-Q system?

Options

    A. Anterior vaginal wall 3 cm proximal to the hymen.
    B. Posterior vaginal wall 3 cm proximal to the hymen.
    C. Most distal edge of the cervix.
    D. Measure from middle of external urethral meatus to anterior midline hymen.
    E. Depth of vagina after point C is reduced to normal position.

204. A 51-year-old para 3 is in your gynaecology clinic for a follow-up appointment with an 8-month history of pelvic pain, urgency and urinary frequency. The pain is sharp in nature, is worse after sexual intercourse and is relieved during voiding. A urinalysis is negative, physical examination is unremarkable and a diary shows frequent, small volume voids. Urodynamics show hypersensitivity during filling cystometry and small bladder capacity. Cystoscopy shows mucosal punctate haemorrhages, and a detrusor muscle biopsy shows an increased mast cell count. She is diagnosed with interstitial cystitis.

Which of the following is administered by instillation in the bladder?

Options

- A. Sodium pentosan polysulphate.
- B. Calcium glycerophosphate.
- C. Hyaluronic acid.
- D. L-arginine.
- E. Amitriptyline.

205. You see a 58-year-old woman in your gynaecology clinic. She has had a vaginal hysterectomy 12 years ago for menorrhagia and now presents with a 6-month history of a lump coming down in the vagina. The lump is uncomfortable during sexual intercourse. She does not have a significant medical history and denies urinary incontinence. On examination a vaginal vault prolapse is identified. She wishes definitive surgical management, and you consent her for an abdominal sacrocolpopexy.

Which of the following is a recognized complication?

Options

- A. Sexual dysfunction.
- B. Posterior vaginal wall prolapse.
- C. Buttock pain.
- D. Shortening of the vagina.
- E. Injury to the internal pudendal artery.

Module 18 Urogynaecology and pelvic floor disorders

ANSWERS

193. Answer: B.

Explanation: The voiding diary (or frequency-volume chart) is a simple but effective tool for assessing storage symptoms. It is helpful in determining the volume of fluid intake, urinary frequency, nocturia, voided volume and any episodes of leakage, and it is recommended in the initial assessment of all women with urinary incontinence.

Reference: National Institute for Health and Care Excellence (2013). Clinical guideline 171. Urinary incontinence in women. London.

194. Answer: A.

Explanation: A Q_{max} of 20 to 36 ml with a postresidual volume less than 100 to 150 ml and maximum cystometric capacity between 300 and 600 ml would be acceptable normal values. Detrusor contractions at this point suggest detrusor overactivity.

Reference: Moore, K (2013). *Urogynaecology: Evidence-Based Clinical Practice*. London: Springer-Verlag.

195. Answer: B.

Explanation: Women with stress or mixed urinary incontinence should be offered a trial of supervised pelvic floor training of at least 3 months' duration as first-line treatment. Pelvic floor muscle training programmes should comprise at least eight contractions performed three times per day.

Reference: National Institute for Health and Care Excellence (2013). Clinical guideline 171. Urinary incontinence in women. London.

196. Answer: D.

Explanation: Generally, 50% of women with mixed urinary incontinence have resolution of urge symptoms, 25% have no change and 25% have a worsening of their symptoms after a midurethral sling procedure.

Reference: Dmochowski, R (2013). *Surgery for Urinary Incontinence: Female Pelvic Surgery Video Atlas Series*. New York: Elsevier Health Sciences.

197. Answer: D.

Explanation: After a multidisciplinary team review, bladder wall injection with botulinum toxin A should be offered to women with overactive bladder (OAB) caused by proven detrusor overactivity that has not responded to conservative management (including OAB drug therapy). Neither transcutaneous posterior tibial nerve nor sacral nerve stimulation should be offered to treat women with OAB.

Reference: National Institute for Health and Care Excellence (2013). Clinical guideline 171. Urinary incontinence in women. London.

198. Answer: C.

Explanation: When offering a synthetic midurethral tape procedure, surgeons should use a device manufactured from type 1 macroporous polypropylene tape, using a bottom-up retropubic approach.

Reference: National Institute for Health and Care Excellence (2013). Clinical guideline 171. Urinary incontinence in women. London.

199. Answer: E.

Explanation: Duloxetine may be offered as second-line therapy if women prefer pharmacologic to surgical treatment or are not suitable for surgical treatment.

Reference: National Institute for Health and Care Excellence (2013). Clinical guideline 171. Urinary incontinence in women. London.

200. Answer: A.

Explanation: Synthetic tapes and slings should not be used in individuals with neurogenic stress incontinence because of the risk of urethral erosion.

Reference: National Institute for Health and Care Excellence (2012). Clinical guideline 148. Management of lower urinary tract dysfunction in neurological disease. London.

201. Answer: C.

Explanation: McCall's culdoplasty at the time of vaginal hysterectomy is a recommended measure to prevent enterocele formation.

Reference: Royal College of Obstetricians and Gynaecologists (2007). Green-top Guideline No. 46. The management of post hysterectomy vaginal vault prolapse. London.

202. Answer: E.

Explanation: Colpocleisis entails closure of the vagina, which is suitable for frail women who do not want to retain sexual function. The procedure can be done under local anaesthetic.

Reference: Royal College of Obstetricians and Gynaecologists (2007). Green-top Guideline No. 46. The management of post hysterectomy vaginal vault prolapse. London.

203. Answer: D.

Explanation: Genital hiatus is measured from the middle of the external urethral meatus to the posterior midline hymen.

Reference: Bump, R. et al. (1996). The standardization of terminology of female pelvic organ prolapse and pelvic floor dysfunction. *American Journal of Obstetrics and Gynecology* 175 (1), 10–17.

204. Answer: C.

Explanation: Hyaluronic acid is licensed for use in the UK. It temporarily replaces the deficient glycosaminoglycan (GAG) layer on the bladder wall, helping to relieve the pain, frequency and urgency of interstitial cystitis. For the first 4 weeks of treatment, women with interstitial cystitis receive one instillation each week. After that, treatments are usually given once a month until the symptoms resolve.

Reference: Jha S, Parsons M (2007). Painful bladder syndrome and interstitial cystitis. *The Obstetrician & Gynaecologist* 9, 34–41.

205. Answer: B.

Explanation: There is increased incidence of posterior vaginal wall prolapse following abdominal sacrocolpopexy.

Reference: Royal College of Obstetricians and Gynaecologists (2007). Green-top Guideline No. 46. The management of post hysterectomy vaginal vault prolapse. London.

Illustrated questions

QUESTIONS

206. A 32-year-old primigravida at 29 weeks' gestation is referred by her community midwife as she is clinically small for dates (SFH is 24 cm). Ultrasound biometry shows an estimated fetal weight below the 10th centile and the UA Doppler image is shown in Figure 206.

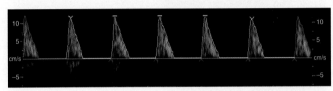

What is the optimal management strategy?

Options

    A. Daily CTG + repeat ultrasound daily for UA Doppler and DV Doppler. Recommend delivery by caesarean section before 32 weeks' gestation after steroids if either the DV Doppler or CTG is abnormal.

    B. Daily CTG + repeat ultrasound daily for UA Doppler and DV Doppler. Recommend delivery by 37 weeks after steroids if either the DV Doppler or CTG is abnormal.

    C. Daily CTG + repeat ultrasound daily for UA Doppler and DV Doppler. Recommend induction of labour before 34 weeks after steroids if either the DV Doppler or CTG is abnormal.

    D. Daily CTG + repeat ultrasound weekly for UA Doppler and DV Doppler. Recommend delivery before 32 weeks after steroids if either the DV Doppler or CTG is abnormal.

    E. Daily CTG + repeat ultrasound daily for MCA Doppler. Recommend delivery before 32 weeks after steroids if either the MCA Doppler or CTG is abnormal.

207. A 70-year-old patient, who is otherwise fit and well, presents with multiple lesions on her vulva extending to her vulva and vagina as shown in Figure 207. A biopsy is reported as basal cell carcinoma and a magnetic resonance image shows right inguinal and femoral lymph node involvement.

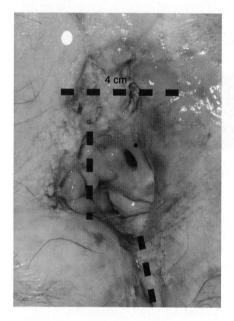

4 cm

What would be the appropriate management?

Options

- A. Radical excision and en-bloc dissection + bilateral nodal dissection.
- B. Radical excision and en-bloc dissection + selective sentinel node excision.
- C. Radical excision and en-bloc dissection + unilateral nodal dissection.
- D. Wide local excision + bilateral nodal dissection.
- E. Wide local excision + unilateral nodal dissection.

208. The pathology demonstrated in Figure 208 may be associated with which of the following scenarios?

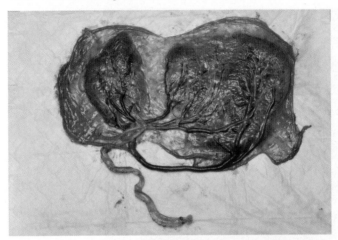

Options

A. Bleeding at the time of spontaneous or artificial rupture of membranes followed by fetal bradycardia.

B. Clear liquor at the time of spontaneous or artificial rupture of membranes preceded by fetal bradycardia.

C. Fetal tachycardia without vaginal bleeding.

D. Abnormal CTG with normal fetal blood sample results.

E. Poor progress of labour requiring a caesarean section.

209. Regarding the abnormality shown in Figure 209, evidence suggests that:

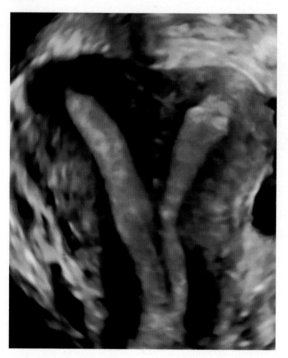

Options

A. Expectant management is recommended in patients with recurrent miscarriage less than 35 years of age.

B. There is a high risk of ectopic pregnancy.

C. Surgical correction is recommended in patients less than 35 years of age with subfertility.

D. Surgical correction is recommended to patients greater than 40 years of age with subfertility.

E. Surgical correction may be beneficial to patients with recurrent miscarriage when no other problem has been identified.

210. A 22-year-old nulliparous patient presents to the surgeons with an episode of postcoital vaginal bleeding 10 days previously and 5 days of increasing right lower abdominal pain. Abdominal and pelvic examinations demonstrate guarding and marked tenderness. Her temperature is 39.2°C, heart rate 102 bpm and BP 110/70 mm Hg. Blood tests show a raised C-reactive protein of 400 mg/L, a WBC of 30.5 × 10⁹/L and a negative pregnancy test. Appendicitis is expected, and you are called to theatre by the surgeons for a gynaecological opinion (Figure 210).

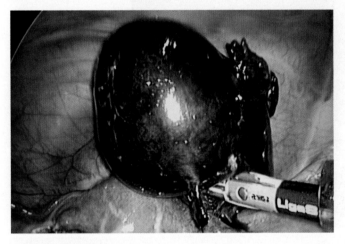

What is your recommendation?

Options

  A. Adnexectomy.
  B. Central oophoropexy.
  C. Detorsion.
  D. Do nothing, as patient is not consented for any procedure on the adnexa.
  E. Lateral oophoropexy.

211. The pathology shown in Figure 211 is associated with which of the following?

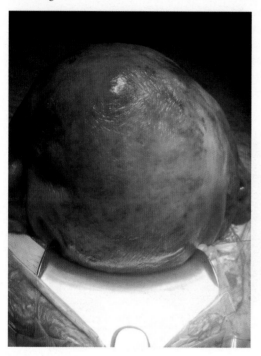

Options

- A. Congenital fetal anomalies.
- B. Placenta praevia.
- C. Placental abruption.
- D. Twin pregnancy.
- E. Vasa praevia.

212. A 30-year-old para 1 presents at 10 weeks' gestation with left-sided lower abdominal pain, dizziness and shoulder-tip pain. There is tenderness in the left adnexa on bimanual examination, and Figure 212 shows the laparoscopic appearances.

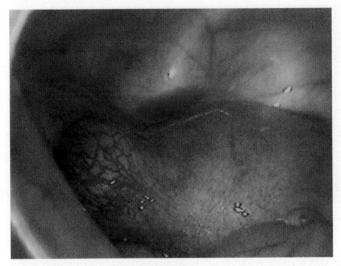

What is the incidence of this condition?

Options

    A. 0.05% of all ectopic pregnancies.
    B. 0.5% of all ectopic pregnancies.
    C. 5% of all ectopic pregnancies.
    D. 10% of all ectopic pregnancies.
    E. 12.5% of all ectopic pregnancies.

213. A 30-year-old patient is diagnosed with Stage IB cervical cancer. She wishes to retain her fertility and undergoes trachelectomy with laparoscopic pelvic lymphadenectomy.

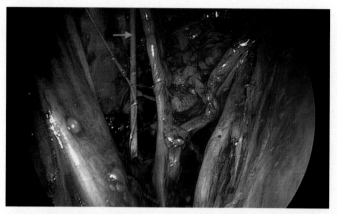

Figure courtesy of Mr Anish Bali, Consultant Gynaecologist/Oncologist Surgeon, Derby Teaching Hospitals NHS Foundation Trust, with permission.

The structure marked in Figure 213 is accidentally cut, which results in:

Options

A. Numbness and paraesthesia on the medial aspect of the thigh and weakness in adduction of the thigh.

B. Numbness and paraesthesia on the lateral aspect of the thigh and weakness in abduction of the thigh.

C. Numbness and paraesthesia on the medial aspect of the thigh and weakness in abduction of the thigh.

D. Numbness and paraesthesia on the lateral aspect of the thigh and weakness in adduction of the thigh.

E. None of the above.

214. This is a filling cystomyogram (Figure 214) of a 56-year-old para 3 who is referred to the urodynamics one-stop clinic.

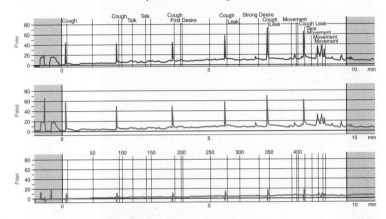

What best describes the findings?

Options

    A. Detrusor overactivity.

    B. Mixed urinary incontinence.

    C. Normal study.

    D. Urodynamic stress incontinence.

    E. Bladder outflow obstruction.

215. This fetal abnormality in Figure 215:

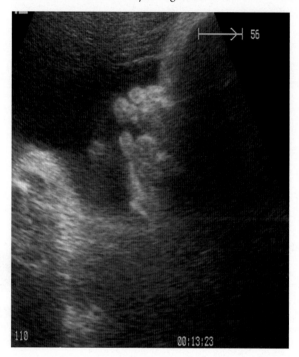

Options

A. Is consistent with a teratoma of branchial origin?
B. Is more commonly midline than lateral?
C. Is associated with tetracycline usage?
D. Has an incidence of around 1:2000?
E. Can be associated with polyhydramnios?

216. What is the perinatal mortality rate associated with this condition (Figure 216)?

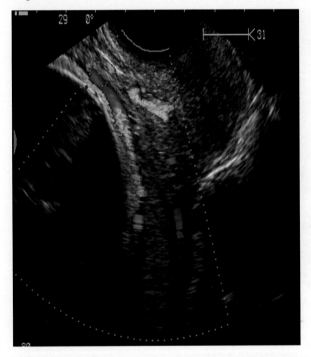

Options

    A. Around 5%.
    B. Around 25%.
    C. Around 40%.
    D. Around 60%.
    E. Around 90%.

217. A 23-year-old primigravida attends for her fetal anomaly scan at 20 weeks' gestation. The image in Figure 217 is seen.

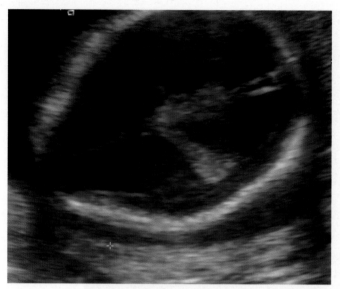

What is the most common mechanism leading to this finding?

Options

    A. Impaired CSF resorption.

    B. Obstruction to flow of CSF.

    C. Overproduction of CSF.

    D. Underdevelopment of cortical tissue.

    E. Ultrasound artefact.

218. A 25-year-old nulliparous woman is delivered by elective caesarean for breech presentation (Figure 218).

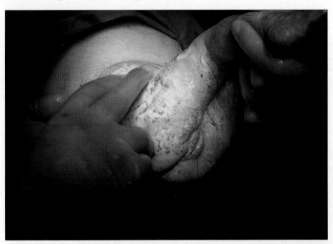

What are the approximate chances of a successful vaginal birth in her next pregnancy?

Options

    A. 65%.
    B. 70%.
    C. 75%.
    D. 80%.
    E. 85%.

219. A 39-year-old primigravida in with an IVF singleton pregnancy is undergoing a detailed ultrasound following a nuchal translucency measurement of 3.2 mm. The four-chamber cardiac view is shown in Figure 219.

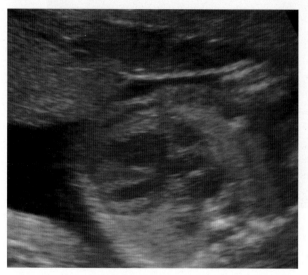

What would be the most appropriate next step?

Options

A. Reassure her that the four chambers have developed symmetrically and that no further action is required.

B. Explain that the right ventricle is larger than the left and that the baby probably has a hypoplastic left heart. The prognosis will be, at best, guarded and termination is worth considering.

C. Point out that the atria are separated by a cystic structure of uncertain origin.

D. Offer fetal genetic studies.

E. Explain that the appearances suggest Fallot's tetralogy and that the duct will need to be kept open with a postnatal prostaglandin infusion.

220. A para 1 with treated hypothyroidism is seen for a scan at 19 weeks' gestation, and Figure 220 is taken. The pregnancy is complicated by impaired glucose tolerance at 22 weeks and a small painless PV bleed 1 week later. When seen for review at 29 weeks, one of the twins is on the 10th centile and the other above the 50th, with an estimated 25% difference in estimated fetal weight. The liquor seems reasonably normal.

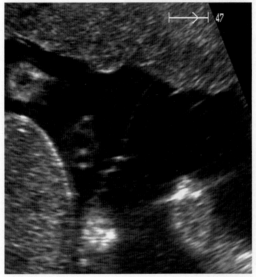

What is your next step?

Options

A. Given the likelihood of TTTS, you give steroids and refer to a fetal medicine centre.

B. Given the fact that the liquor seems reasonably normal around each, you feel that TTTS is unlikely and arrange a 2-week review.

C. Given that the bladder of the smaller twin is not visualized when checked, the staging is Quintero II.

D. Given that there is 25% difference in estimated fetal weights, you decide to undertake Doppler studies for placental dysfunction.

E. Given that there is 25% difference in estimated fetal weights, you are concerned about chromosomal abnormality and broach the subject of amniocentesis.

221. You are called to the postnatal ward to see a 37-year-old para 3 who, after a reasonably long induced labour, has had a vaginal delivery 3 hours previously (Figure 221).

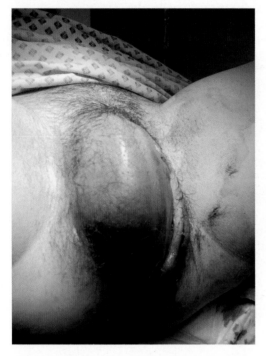

What would be the most reasonable course of action?

Options

    A. Given the risks of bleeding after releasing the tamponade, you recommend tight support briefs and review the following day.

    B. Transfer to theatre for incision and drainage under general anaesthesia.

    C. Given the possibility of extension to the broad ligament, you arrange a computed tomography scan of the pelvis.

    D. Incision and drainage under local anaesthetic.

    E. Concerned about pressure on the femoral vein, you start prophylactic subcutaneous heparin.

222. A 35-year-old para 0 + 0 with a BMI of 26 is seen after her 20-week fetal anatomy scan. The fetal anatomy is normal, but a uterine artery Doppler is performed (Figure 222).

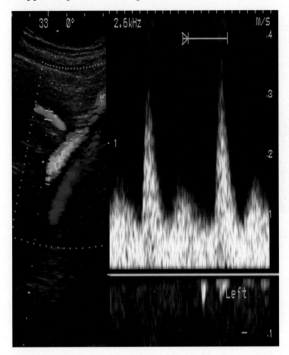

What would be the most appropriate action?

Options

    A. Assessment of fetal size and umbilical artery Doppler in third trimester.

    B. Repeat uterine artery Doppler at 24 weeks.

    C. Serial assessment of fetal size and umbilical artery Doppler from 24 to 26 weeks.

    D. Serial assessment of fetal size and umbilical artery Doppler from 26 to 28 weeks.

    E. Serial assessment of fetal size from 28 weeks.

223. You are asked to attend an obstetric emergency call for the problem shown in Figure 223. The midwives successfully manage the problem, and you then advise them to prepare for PPH.

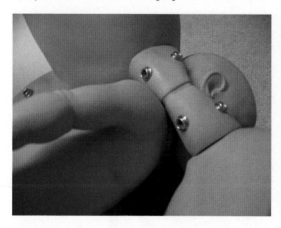

What is the approximate chance of PPH?

Options

    A. 2%.
    B. 5%.
    C. 10%.
    D. 20%.
    E. 30%.

224. With regard to the scenario depicted in Figure 223:

Options

    A. Early induction of labour is a reasonable course of action to minimize the risk of complications in all those with an estimated fetal weight greater than 4.5 kg.
    B. McRoberts' manoeuvre before delivery of the head is helpful in preventing the scenario.
    C. Caesarean prevents brachial plexus injury.
    D. Fundal pressure should only be applied when suprapubic pressure is used to guard the lower segment.
    E. The incidence is between 0.5 and 0.7%.

Illustrated questions

ANSWERS

206. Answer: A.

Explanation: In a preterm SGA fetus with absent end diastolic flow detected before 32 weeks of gestation, delivery is recommended when the DV Doppler becomes abnormal or umbilical vein pulsations appear, and after completion of steroids. Even when venous Doppler is normal, delivery is recommended by 32 weeks of gestation and should be considered between 30 and 32 weeks of gestation. In a preterm SGA fetus, MCA Doppler has limited ability to predict acidaemia or adverse outcome, and should not be used to time delivery.

Reference: Royal College of Obstetricians and Gynaecologists (2014). Green-top Guideline No. 31. The investigation and management of the small-for-gestational-age fetus, 2nd ed. London.

207. Answer: A.

Explanation: The lesion shown in the image is multifocal with the main ulcerating area involving the anterior vulva in the midline, as well as the lower urethra and vagina. Radiology suggests probable lymph node involvement, and it is therefore likely to be at least Stage III. Unilateral dissection is appropriate for lesions up to 4 cm in diameter that are at least 1 cm from the midline, as long as the unilateral nodes are negative. Lesions involving the anterior labia should have bilateral dissection because of the more frequent contralateral lymphatic drainage from this region. In unifocal tumours of less than 4 cm in maximum diameter where there is no clinical suspicion of lymph node involvement, patients can be safely managed by removal of the identified sentinel lymph nodes.

Reference: Royal College of Obstetricians and Gynaecologists (2014). Guidelines for the diagnosis and management of vulval carcinoma. London.

208. Answer: A.

Explanation: The image shows a bilobed placenta structure, marginal insertion of umbilical cord and partial velamentous insertions of cord (fetal vessels traversing the membranes to reach the smaller placental lobe on the right). The reported incidence varies between one in 2000 and one in 6000 pregnancies.

Reference: Royal College of Obstetricians and Gynaecologists (2011). Green-top Guideline No. 27. Placenta Praevia, placenta praevia accreta and vasa praevia: Diagnosis and management. London.

209. Answer: E.

Explanation: Although the usefulness of septoplasty has yet to be established, an RCT has been published that compared septoplasty performed using a bipolar Versapoint™ electrode (Ethicon Gynecare, Johnson & Johnson Medical Ltd., Livingston, UK; 5-mm telescope) with that performed using a monopolar electrode (8-mm telescope) in 161 women with a septate uterus and a history of recurrent miscarriage or primary subfertility. There was no difference in pregnancy rates between the two groups. A reanalysis of the original data showed that treatment was less beneficial to women with subfertility than to those with recurrent miscarriage. Nonrandomized controlled trials have shown that hysteroscopic septoplasty improves natural conception rates in women with otherwise unexplained subfertility, as well as the success of women undergoing IVF treatment.

Reference: Colacurci N, De Franciscis P, Mollo A, Litta P, Perino A, Cobellis L, et al. (2007). Small-diameter hysteroscopy with Versapoint versus resectoscopy with a unipolar knife for the treatment of septate uterus: a prospective randomized study. *Journal of Minimally Invasive Gynecology* 14, 622–627.

210. Answer: A.

Explanation: This is an adnexal torsion; the blue-black appearances may be caused by lymphatic and venous stasis rather than arterial ischaemia. Untwisting is an option and might eventually result in functioning ovarian tissue, but success decreases with time and symptoms have been present for greater than 48 hours. Furthermore, there is a marked systemic inflammatory response and leaving such a necrotic-looking adnexal lesion might lead to systemic deterioration. On balance, removal is probably the most appropriate way forward.

Reference: Damigos E, Johns J, Ross J (2012). An update on the diagnosis and management of ovarian torsion. *The Obstetrician & Gynaecologist* 14, 229–236.

211. Answer: C.

Explanation: The image shows a Couvelaire uterus. It is caused when haemorrhage from placental blood vessels causes placental separation, followed by blood infiltration in the myometrium.

Reference: Habek D, Selthofer R, Kulas T (2008). Uteroplacental apoplexy (Couvelaire syndrome). *Wiener Klinische Wochenschrift* 120, 88.

212. Answer C.

Explanation: Interstitial pregnancy accounts for between 1% and 6% of all ectopic pregnancies.

Reference: Jermy K, et al. (2004) The conservative management of interstitial pregnancy. *BJOG* 111 (11), 1283–1288.

213. Answer: A.

Explanation: Injury of the obturator nerve results in numbness and paraesthesia on the medial aspect of the thigh and weakness in adduction of the thigh.

Reference: Sinnatamby, CS (2011). *Last's Anatomy: Regional and Applied.* Amsterdam: Elsevier Health Sciences.

214. Answer: D.

Explanation: This study shows urodynamic stress incontinence. Urine leak is observed on coughing and changing position. The detrusor muscle remained stable.

Reference: Abrams PR (2006). *Urodynamics.* New York: Springer.

215. Answer: E.

Explanation: Cleft lip has an incidence of approximately 1 : 700. They are more commonly unilateral or bilateral rather than midline, and may be associated with polyhydramnios if swallowing is difficult. Tetracylines can cause staining of the teeth and enamel hypoplasia, but not cleft lip.

Reference: Dixon MJ, et al. (2011). Cleft lip and palate: understanding genetic and environmental influences. *Nature Reviews Genetics* 12 (3), 167–178.

216. Answer: D.

Explanation: Vasa praevia describes fetal vessels coursing through the membranes over the internal cervical os and below the fetal presenting part, unprotected by placental tissue or umbilical cord. It often presents with fresh vaginal bleeding at the time of membrane rupture and fetal heart abnormalities such as decelerations, bradycardia and sinusoidal trace or fetal demise. The mortality rate in this situation is around 60%. The survival rate is up to 97% when diagnosis has been made antenatally.

Reference: Royal College of Obstetricians and Gynaecologists (2011). Green-top Guideline No. 27. Placenta praevia, placenta praevia accreta and vasa praevia: Diagnosis and management. London.

217. Answer: B.

Explanation: This is hydrocephalus. Obstruction to the flow of CSF could be aqueduct stenosis, which can be associated with infection, genetic abnormality, mass lesions or bleeding.

Reference: Cameron A, et al. (2011). *Fetal Medicine for the MRCOG and Beyond*. London: RCOG Press, 61–62.

218. Answer: E.

Explanation: The chance of successful vaginal birth after an elective caesarean section for malpresentation is 84%.

Reference: Royal College of Obstetricians and Gynaecologists (2015). Green-top Guideline No 45. Birth after previous caesarean birth, 2nd ed. London.

219. Answer: E.

Explanation: This is Fallot's tetralogy: the aorta is overriding the ventricular septum and there is a marked ventriculoseptal defect. Although it is associated with chromosomal abnormality, explanation of the condition should come before chromosomal testing. Unlike with transposition of the great vessels, however, immediate postnatal management does not require ductal patency to be maintained.

220. Answer: D.

Explanation: The T sign in this image is consistent with a monochorionic diamniotic twin pregnancy. Although there is a risk of TTTS, this is unlikely here because there is no oligohydramnios/polyhydramnios sequence, and a single check of the bladder is insufficient to make a statement about its absence. Even if the bladder was absent, the Quintero Staging would be I, with abnormal Dopplers being required for Stage II. Being monochorionic, it is very likely that both twins are genetically identical and amniocentesis may risk preterm labour. Doppler studies to look for placental dysfunction seem most appropriate.

Reference: National Institute for Health and Care Excellence (2011). Guideline 129. Multiple pregnancy: The management of twin and triplet pregnancies in the antenatal period. London.

221. Answer: B.

Explanation: Conservative management for vulval haematoma is not unreasonable, but this patient carries two risk factors for postnatal VTE (age > 35 years, and para 3), so prophylactic subcutaneous heparin is indicated, yet cannot be given with such a substantial haematoma. Conservative management also risks infection. It is very likely that the haematoma is deep, and local anaesthesia would be inadequate to allow the cavity to be sutured closed.

Reference: Royal College of Obstetricians and Gynaecologists (2015). Green-top Guideline No 37a. Reducing the risk of venous thromboembolism during pregnancy and the puerperium. London.

222. Answer: D.

Explanation: This woman has three minor risk factors for an SGA fetus (BMI greater than 25, age 35, nulliparity), and it has been for these reasons that a uterine artery Doppler has been assessed. It shows notching, and the fetus is therefore at increased risk of SGA.

Reference: Royal College of Obstetricians and Gynaecologists (2013). Green-top Guideline No. 31. Small for gestational age, 2nd ed. London.

223. Answer: C.

Explanation: The risk of PPH after shoulder dystocia is 11%.

Reference: Royal College of Obstetricians and Gynaecologists (2012). Green-top Guideline No. 42. Shoulder dystocia, 2nd ed. London.

224. Answer: E.

Explanation: This image depicts shoulder dystocia. Induction of labour is only warranted in those with impaired glucose tolerance; there is no evidence that it is helpful otherwise. McRoberts' position does not prevent shoulder dystocia from occurring, but it is very useful in management. Four percent of brachial plexus injuries are following a caesarean section rather than vaginal delivery; and fundal pressure should never be applied.

Reference: Royal College of Obstetricians and Gynaecologists (2012). Green-top Guidelines No. 42. Shoulder dystocia, 2nd ed. London.

Index

Page numbers followed by "*f*" indicate figures.